"Q-Tip is gone," ▓▓▓▓▓▓▓▓▓▓▓▓▓▓▓▓ revamping Dacron's wardrobe, ▓▓▓▓▓▓▓▓▓▓▓"

"Where is Dacron?" Ricardo asked.

As if on cue, the door from the hallway swung open, and Dacron jumped into the room. Gone was his minimalist hairdo; in its place was a dramatic mane. A cluster of gold chains glittered at his neck. The top three buttons of his shirt collar were unbuttoned, revealing a shock of chest hair that hadn't been there yesterday, and the back of his collar was turned up rakishly. The rhinestones on his hiphuggers caught the light.

"Thangyouvurymuch," he said as he grasped the micro-phone, rings glistening on every finger. "Ah wanna do a little number for yuh now that ah think you'll like."

Without a doubt, here was a different Dacron than the one the crew had been used to. Among androids, now he was clearly The King....

STAR WRECK V
The Undiscovered Nursing Home
A PARODY

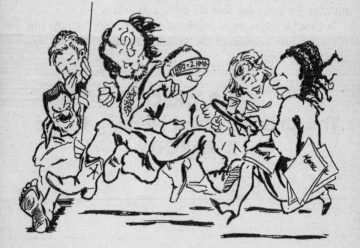

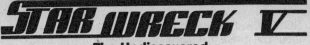

STAR WRECK V

The Undiscovered Nursing Home

An intergalactic gaggle of guffaws

by

LEAH REWOLINSKI

ILLUSTRATIONS BY
HARRY TRUMBORE

A 2M COMMUNICATIONS LTD. PRODUCTION

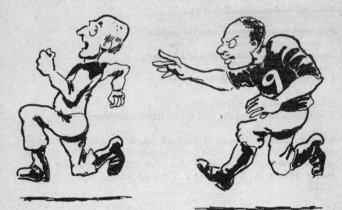

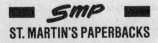

SMP

ST. MARTIN'S PAPERBACKS

NOTE: If you purchased this book without a cover you should be aware that this book is stolen property. It was reported as "unsold and destroyed" to the publisher, and neither the author nor the publisher has received any payment for this "stripped book."

Star Wreck is an unauthorized parody of the *Star Trek* television and motion picture series, the *Star Trek: The Next Generation* television series, and the *Star Trek: Deep Space Nine* television series. None of the individuals or companies associated with these series or with any merchandise based upon these series, has in any way sponsored, approved, endorsed or authorized this book.

Published by arrangement with the author

STAR WRECK V: THE UNDISCOVERED NURSING HOME

Copyright © 1993 by Leah Rewolinski.

Cover illustration by Bob Larkin.
Text illustrations copyright © 1993 by Harry Trumbore.

All rights reserved. No part of this book may be used or reproduced in any manner whatsoever without written permission except in the case of brief quotations embodied in critical articles or reviews. For information address St. Martin's Press, 175 Fifth Avenue, New York, N.Y. 10010.

ISBN: 0-312-95122-1

Printed in the United States of America

St. Martin's Paperbacks edition/September 1993

10 9 8 7 6 5 4 3 2 1

To Tom, the undiscovered CPA

Contents

1

Do Not Go Gently Into That Good Riddance

CAPT. JAMES T. SMIRK studied his reflection in the mirror. *Still smashing after all these years*, he decided. Then he felt a sharp tug at the back of his scalp.

"Ouch!" Smirk exclaimed, rising reflexively a few inches out of the chair.

"Oops. Sorry, Captain," the barber said. "Guess I got a little carried away. But you did say you were in a hurry."

As Smirk warily settled down in the chair again, the barber carefully lifted another strand of the hairpiece and continued tightening the weave that held it to Smirk's own hair.

"*I am* in a hurry, Mr. Seville," Smirk replied. "I've got a meeting with a Starfreak admiral in half an hour. But can't you work fast without scalping me?"

"It'll be done in a few minutes," the barber soothed him. "We want it to look natural, don't we?"

"Absolutely," Smirk replied, checking his reflection again. *I must admit*, he thought, *I've aged better than any of my crew*. He began imagining the others from the USS *Endocrine* who were waiting here with him at Starfreak Headquarters.

Take Mr. Smock, for instance. His permanently dour expression had hardened into a chiseled mask that made him a prime candidate for the fifth face on Mt. Rushmore. And though Smock's Vulture eyebrows maintained their youthful tilt, everyone knew he achieved this facelift illusion with cellophane tape strategically placed beneath his bangs.

Zulu had started to take on the serenity of an ancient Zen

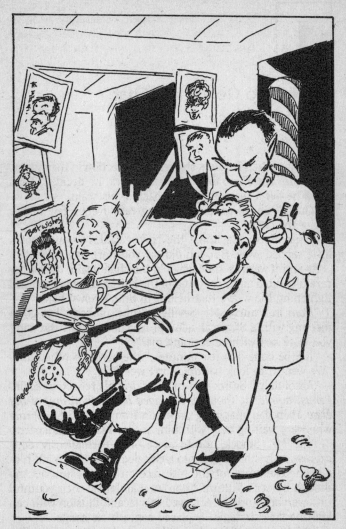

I must admit, Smirk thought, I've aged better than any of my crew.

master. But Smirk had never thought of serenity as an essential quality for a Starfreak officer, especially when it meant, as in Zulu's case, taking several four-hour naps every day.

Checkout's boyish features clashed with the wrinkles he'd acquired. His behavior embodied the expression "There's no fool like an old fool," and often he smelled of Ben Gay.

As for Chief Engineer Snot, it was a contest to see which was drooping faster—his jowls, his chins, or his pot belly.

Dr. McCaw had been a lot more spry lately; rumor had it that he'd given himself a hip replacement without telling anyone. Still, there were years of crankiness etched into his face, and he complained that the bursitis in his shoulder was a serious hindrance to his medical practice because it affected his golf swing.

Then there was Yoohoo, Smirk's communications officer, who seemed to have frosted her hair with typewriter correction fluid. Yoohoo had adopted the annoying habit of lecturing young Starfreak recruits on how easy they had it nowadays. "In the old days all this electronic equipment was manually operated," she often pointed out. "It took six strong crewmembers to hold open the shuttlebay doors. And the vacuum sucking them out into space was a lot stronger then, too."

And despite his unquenchable confidence in his own appearance, Smirk himself had the uneasy suspicion that there was a Starfreak conspiracy afoot to convince him to step aside and let some young punk take his place. The conspirators had even gone so far as to sell his name to a mailing list for the elderly. At least, that was Smirk's explanation for why his mail these days consisted mostly of catalogs offering liver spot creme and subscriptions to *Senility Digest*.

Smirk thought, *Well, they can hint all they want. We're not stepping aside until we're good and ready. We're not getting older, we're getting bitter. Er, better.*

Smirk's mind ambled back to the present; the barber had finished tightening his hairpiece and was now styling it. As he pulled a miniature rake through the top to create height, the barber said, "You might want to try a new look one of these days, Captain. Astroturf is really hot right now. Once we weave a patch of that onto the back of your head, we can carve into it anything you want: your initials, a gang insignia, whatever." Expertly he wielded a curling iron to touch up the waves on either side of Smirk's crown.

"No thanks, Mr. Seville. I'll stick with the old tried and true," Smirk replied. "It seems to work pretty well with the ladies," he added, his voice straining with false modesty.

"You sure you won't try it?" Seville asked, grinning at Smirk in the mirror. "We could carve some sweetheart's initials into the 'turf—whoever your latest conquest is at the moment."

Smirk returned the grin. "Heck," he retorted, "I'd be in here every few hours for a re-carving—the initials would change too often."

Seville chuckled. "Just trying to drum up business," he said, putting the finishing touches on the curl that drooped fetchingly over Smirk's forehead.

As Smirk headed down the crowded hallway from the barber shop to the admirals' offices, his mind meandered pleasantly between speculation and observation.

It's odd that they wouldn't tell me which admiral I'd be meeting with, he thought. *They just said that it would be "whoever is on call at the time." Whatever happened to protocol?*

Wow, look at that hot mama. She's the one I put the moves on at the singles' dance last night. She's looking my way. She likes the hair, I can tell.

Maybe the admiral wants to apologize for the way Star-freak Command treated us after we lost the Fountain of Youth to the Romanumens. Sure, it meant a couple quadzillion dollars in potential profit down the drain, but did that justify threatening to throw both Endocrine *crews out of the fleet? Good thing Captain Ricardo's bartender used her stash of fountain water to bargain with Starfreak and get back our commissions.*

Hey, there's that little filly who offered to read my palm during breakfast this morning. An old ploy, but a good one. I'll give her the look that says I'd love to stop and chat if only I weren't on my way to an important meeting.

Maybe Starfreak wants to tell me that they've finished the thirty-zillion-mile tuneup on my ship, and they're giving us a new mission.

Oh, man, there's that bouncy little ensign. She looks even better in her Starfreak uniform than she did in her bikini at the pool yesterday. Ahhh, if only I could be a strand of Lycra on her tunic for a minute—oooh, baby!

The distractions made Smirk wonder just how many classy dames were staying here at Starfreak Headquarters at the moment. *There must be at least two thousand or so,* he thought. *And I've gone through nearly all of them. It's been a busy week. Time to get back into the field for some new life forms.*

In the waiting room of the admirals' office area, a light flashed at the receptionist's console. He consulted the readout, then turned to Smirk and told him, "The admiral will see you now."

"Thanks," Smirk replied, setting aside the copy of *U.S. News & Universe Report* he'd been reading. He usually preferred to spend his waiting time flirting with the receptionist rather than leafing through old magazines, but seeing a male behind the desk had squelched that idea. *I wonder if they placed a guy there just to make me ill at ease,* he thought.

Smirk relaxed, though, as he entered the office. Although the back of the admiral's chair faced the doorway as its occupant stared out the window, Smirk could see that the admiral was a woman. Suddenly he felt he was back on familiar territory. Whatever this meeting was about, he certainly could charm his way through it. He sat down in the single chair that faced the desk.

Then the admiral swiveled toward him, and Smirk gasped in dismay. He realized this was someone he hadn't seen since the night he'd stood her up for a date. That was a couple of decades ago, but he hadn't forgotten—and from the look on her face, neither had she.

Smirk even recalled the circumstances of that evening long ago. On the way to pick her up for the date, he'd happened upon a stranger—an alien woman with a most extraordinary trio of mammary glands. Smirk, agog with scientific curiosity, had spent the night pursuing the alien instead.

The woman he'd stood up had been a mere lieutenant then. Now, here she was, an admiral who not only outranked him but also seemed intent on outstaring him. He stammered, "A-A-Admiral Less. How good to see you."

She met his eyes with an icy gaze. "You're twenty years, sixteen days, five hours and ten minutes late, Smirk."

"Ah, Ruth," he replied, "still dwelling on our near-date, eh? Let me explain—"

"Never mind." She tapped her five-inch red-lacquered fingernails on the glossy varnish of the desktop. Smirk wondered, *Am I seeing things, or is the nail of her index finger filed to a point?*

"I'm so glad I happened to draw personnel duty today, Captain," Admiral Less continued. "How amusing it is that I'll be the one to break the news to you."

Smirk's hands tightened on the armrests of the chair. *What news?* he wondered.

Obviously savoring the suspense, Admiral Less reached for the pile of mail on her desk, picked up the top envelope, and slit it open with her pointed fingernail. "Mmmmf," she said with a grimace, glancing at the contents. "More junk mail." She tossed the letter into the wastebasket and reached for another.

"Uh, Admiral," Smirk ventured, "you were going to tell me something?"

"Hmmm?" she replied with studied casualness. "Oh, yes." Briskly she straightened up in her chair. Her eyelids narrowed, and the corners of her mouth tilted dangerously upward into unfamiliar smile territory. "Captain, it has come

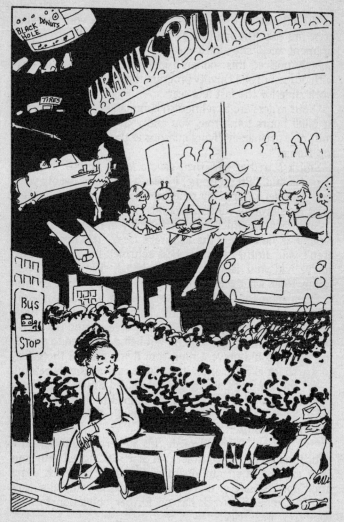

The woman he'd stood up had been a mere lieutenant then.

to the attention of Starfreak Command that you and your crew are past the mandatory retirement age. *Well* past retirement age," she added meanly. "In fact, it's strange that nobody noticed this sooner. I guess we've all been so busy with our new Total Quality program that we've let our regular work slide for the last few years.

"Your orders are to relinquish command of the *Endocrine*. At 0800 hours tomorrow, you and your crew will report to your new permanent living quarters at the Vacant Attic Nursing Home."

Smirk stared at her, then gave a feeble laugh. "Uh-huh. Yes," he said. "Pretty ironic. I break a date, and twenty years later you get revenge by relieving me of command. I guess what goes around comes aground, eh?"

Smirk's grin, which was pretty sickly to begin with, faded rapidly as he studied the admiral's face. "You *are* kidding, aren't you, Ruth?" Admiral Less returned his stare. "Okay, you've had your laugh," Smirk babbled. "We're even. Very funny. Now, what was it you really wanted to see me about?"

For a moment he had a ghastly vision of the mandatory retirement that Less was talking about. Not only would there be the numbing boredom he'd discovered during his crew's previous, voluntary retirement, but being confined to a nursing home would prevent him from flying around the galaxy to search for classy dames. It would be excruciatingly painful.

Yet the admiral's steady gaze shredded Smirk's last hope that this was all a bad joke. He slumped back in the chair. "You're not kidding," he gasped, as though she'd just punched him in the stomach.

"No, I'm not," she affirmed. "It's all very straightforward. Your time is up. The contract that Starfreak signed with your crew expired when our hoard of Fountain of Youth water dried up. The sale of that water was paying your bills. Now that it's gone, Starfreak has no further obligation to keep your crew in service."

A mixture of strong emotions swirled over Smirk's face like an oil slick floating on a puddle. He seemed to waver between punching the admiral in the nose and throwing up on her desk.

"I'm sure you'll like it at the nursing home, Captain," Admiral Less purred with counterfeit pity. "The women outnumber the men five to one."

Then she reached out with one exquisitely manicured fingernail and pressed a button on her desk. A trap door opened beneath Smirk's chair, and he plunged down into darkness.

That night in the ballroom of Starfreak Headquarters, there was a retirement party for Capt. Smirk and his crew. Guests began arriving early, anticipating an evening of boisterous merrymaking.

Starfreak, mindful of Smirk's popularity among the rank and file, had spared no expense for this gala event. The Jell-O molds contained real fruit, there were mountains of Twinkies and HoHos on the buffet, and the Gatorade flowed freely. The room was festooned with genuine balloons and party streamers, not the usual holographic decorations.

Guests admired a display case holding the gold phasers, each engraved with the message "In gratitude for years of faithful service," which the retirees would receive during the ceremony that evening. Most guests were too polite to mention that phasers were inappropriate gifts for officers whose biggest fights in the upcoming years would be waged over who got the best chair in the TV lounge of the nursing home.

Soon after the deejay started playing the first disco number of the evening, the head honchos of Starfreak filed in, signaling the start of the official ceremony. The house lights dimmed, the crowd gathered round, and excitement filled the air. There was just one thing missing: the guests of honor.

At the moment, those guests of honor were down in Starfreak's repair dock, attempting to steal their own ship.

"Are you almost done, Snotty?" Capt. Smirk asked urgently. He stared at Snot's legs and kilt; the rest of the ample

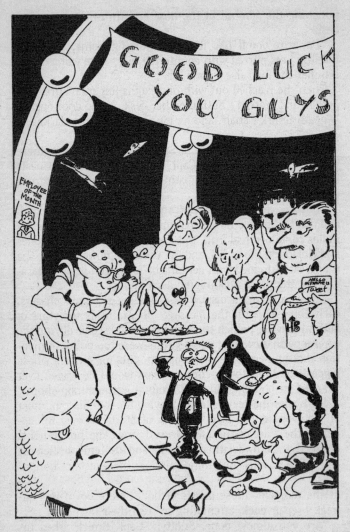

Guests began arriving early.

chief engineer was wedged into the confines of the ship's engine. Smirk added, "How long till you get it started?"

Snot's voice, cranky and strained, emerged from the bowels of the *Endocrine*'s Dilithium Crystal Vanish chamber. "I'm havin' a divvil of a time w' it, Cap'n! This is delicate worrrrk!"

Smirk looked nervously over his shoulder. Most everyone in the repair dock had already left for the retirement party, but someone could have lagged behind and might yet discover them. And though Mr. Smock was posted at the ship's main entrance to intercept anybody who got nosy, Smirk feared that Smock might very well fall asleep on the job. Like Zulu, Smock had become adept at napping.

"Hurry up, Snotty!" Smirk urged. "The tuneup work was already done by Starfreak's mechanics. All you have to do is get the engine to turn over."

"I know, sir," barked Mr. Snot, "but it's not all that easy. It's been a while since I've had t' hot-wire my own ship."

Finally the engine started. Snot had once again conquered the intricacies of matter/antimatter mechanics with a few random, frustrated swipes of his wrench, as well as snarls of Gaelic phrases not found in any tourist guidebook.

Relieved to hear the pulsing of the engine, Smirk rushed to the Bridge. Zulu, Checkout and Yoohoo had already taken their regular stations. Presumably, Dr. McCaw was off brooding in Sick Bay. Mr. Smock, seeing that everything was ready, closed the outer door and turned the deadbolt lock.

Smirk sat in his captain's chair. "Ready for takeoff, Mr. Zulu?" he inquired.

"All systems go," Zulu responded.

"Captain," Mr. Smock broke in, "may I remind you that once we begin the unauthorized use of the ship, there is no turning back."

"No turning back? Tough!" Smirk replied. "What's to turn back to? A life of card games and day outings to the mall? C'mon, Smock, get with it!"

"I support your plan wholeheartedly, Captain," Smock said. "I simply felt it was my duty to point out the consequences."

"Phooey on the consequences! Full speed ahead!" Smirk ordered.

"Moving ahead at impulsive speed," Zulu answered. He pressed the controls, and the ship moved forward in the huge docking bay.

"From now on," Smirk said, increasingly excited now that their venture had officially begun, "I don't want to hear any second thoughts, understand? If you can't go boldly, you shouldn't go at all."

"Captain—" said Mr. Smock.

"No, Smock," interrupted Capt. Smirk, "I don't want any more 'logical' reasons for staying behind."

"Sir—" Smock ventured.

"I mean it," Smirk snapped, swiveling to face him. "No regrets. No more pandering to the brass at headquarters. It's all on our shoulders now, so let's live up to it bravely."

"Captain," Smock said more forcefully, "I am merely trying to tell you that we are headed for the locked doors of the repair bay."

Smirk turned toward the Viewscreen at the front of the Bridge. "Aaaiiy!" he cried. "Where's the door opener? Checkout, isn't this your job?"

"No, Keptin," Checkout replied. "I tink my official duty during takeoff is to fold and sort da road maps."

"Who's got the opener?" demanded Smirk. Checkout and Yoohoo scrambled around the Bridge in a befuddled search for the remote door opener unit, checking the hope chest, the piano bench, and the laundry bin. Meanwhile, the doors loomed ever closer.

"All stop, Mr. Zulu," ordered Smirk.

Zulu stabbed the buttons of his console in vain. "The engines won't respond," he answered. " 'Stop' mode is inoperable, Captain."

"Then throw it in reverse," Smirk suggested. Zulu tried, but that gear was not working either.

"Mr. Snot!" Smirk barked to the intercom. "We need to stop until we can get the bay doors open. Can you give us reverse gear or stop mode? Sometime in the next ten seconds?"

"What?!" Snot yelped over the intercom. "I thought ye wanted t' get out o' here, so I worked like th' dickens t' get ye some forward speeds. W' all due respect, Cap'n, I wish ye would make up yourrr mind!"

"Oh, good grief," Smirk muttered, angry at himself for forgetting that asking Snot to hurry was like asking a glacier to run the 100-meter dash. They'd just wasted a few more precious seconds, and now the doors loomed so close that they filled the entire Viewscreen.

Suddenly Mr. Smock, who'd been staring at the Viewscreen all along, took several long strides toward it. He reached upward and pulled down the sun visor flap at the Viewscreen's top edge. There, fastened to the visor with a loop of wire, was the door opener. Smock pressed its button, and the doors to the repair bay slid open. As the hatch widened, the *Endocrine* slipped out with only inches to spare.

Capt. Smirk exhaled in relief. "Nice work, Mr. Smock," he said. Smock acknowledged the praise with a nod.

"Let's get going before they realize we've left," Smirk continued. "Mr. Zulu, lay in a course for that planet in the Hydrant Quadrant where the Romanumens have claimed the Fountain of Youth. And punch our speed up to Warped Ten."

Mr. Smock regarded Capt. Smirk with his patented raised-eyebrow expression of surprise. "The Fountain of Youth, Captain? Do you have a plan in mind?"

Smirk smiled. "Do I have a plan, Smock?" he chirped. "Have you ever known me *not* to have something up my sleeve? Of course I've got a plan. Now all we have to do is convince the Romanumens to cooperate with it." Smock started to shake his head disapprovingly, but Smirk stopped him with a quick gesture and a smile. "Uh-uh, Mr. Smock," he said. "We're going boldly, remember? Just like in our creed."

As the ship blasted away from Starfreak Headquarters into the vastness beyond, Smirk intoned that creed:

"Space. We need more of it. These are the voyages of the Starship *Endocrine*. Its continuing mission: to cruise around the universe looking for novel predicaments to get into. To search the outskirts of the galaxy for classy dames. To boldly go where nobody wanted to go before!"

Here We Go
A-Dithering

"**G**OOD MORNING, and welcome to our seminar, 'The Politically Correct Starship.' "

As the keynote speaker began, Capt. Jean-Lucy Ricardo leaned forward eagerly, intent on catching every word. However, his crewmembers, seated around him in this crowd at the Starfreak Headquarters lecture hall, were considerably less enthusiastic.

First Officer Wilson Piker was already nodding off. Next to him, Chief Engineer Georgie LaForgery closed the slats of his visor and flicked a switch that would pick up a satellite-TV signal. The others sat moping in varying degrees of boredom.

The crewmembers had reunited more or less by default. Though Starfreak had given back their ship at the end of their previous mission, instead of sticking together, they'd gone their separate ways. However, none of their ventures had worked out as planned.

Dacron the android and Counselor Deanna "Dee" Troit had moved to Milwaukee for a while, but although Dacron enjoyed his job with the Ready Reference Service of the Milwaukee Public Library, the Wisconsin weather didn't agree with him. It had been an especially cold winter. Several times, Deanna needed to call AAA for an emergency jump-start just to enable Dacron to get out of bed.

For her part, Deanna found that leisure activities made it hard to concentrate on her newly established private coun-

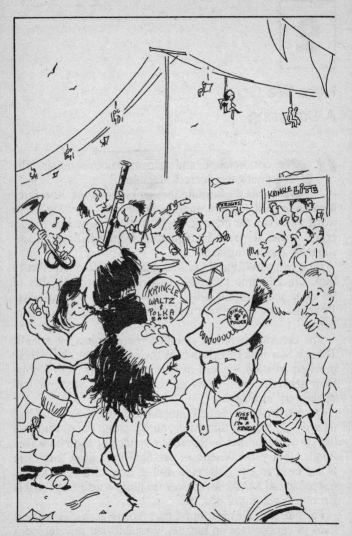

There were just so many festivals to attend....

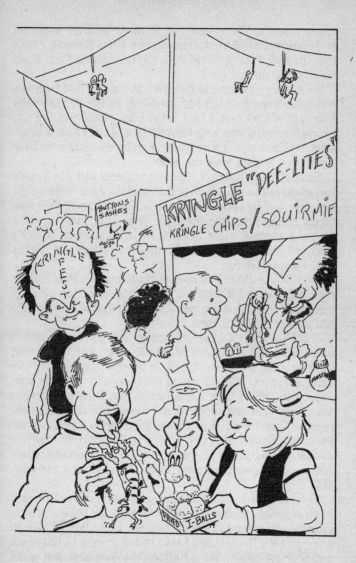

seling practice. There were just so many festivals to attend
on Milwaukee's lakefront: Summerfest, Festa Italiana, Polish
Fest, Kringle Fest, Android Fest, Sentient Being Fest, Festa
Nebula, and on and on.

Even more upsetting to Deanna was the fact that Dacron's
romantic interest in her had vanished. As the effects of the
Fountain of Love water he'd fallen into started wearing off,
his nightly refrain became "Not tonight, dear; I have a head-
ache." Deanna wasn't sure whether androids could even have
headaches, but she took the hint.

Similarly, Dr. Beverage Flusher's romance with Mr. Smock
had sputtered as the effects of the fountain water wore off for
him, too, and he became his old rational self again. Beverage
finally realized that the thrill was gone after they'd spent a
beautiful moonlit night freezing their buns off in Smock's
backyard observatory shed, charting the course of a distant
star, Fossideedee-5.

First Officer Piker had opened his Kringle-cuisine restaurant, mismanaged it for a few months, then left town during
a Board of Health inquiry into the charge that several patrons
had died of food poisoning.

Chief Bartender Guano still had her small private hoard of
water from the Fountains of Truth, Love, and Youth. But
little by little, she'd had to sell off most of the water to pay
living expenses. She was saving the remainder for a dry day.

Security Officer Wart had pulled his son, Smartalecsander,
out of day care and spent several months being a full-time
parent. That led to Wart's hospitalization for nervous ex-
haustion. Smartalecsander was now enrolled in daytime
classes and nighttime activities, and Wart was under doctor's
orders never again to attempt 24-hour custody of a five-year-
old.

Chief Engineer Georgie LaForgery had immersed himself
in an ongoing HolidayDeck program with the computer's re-
creation of a charming fellow engineer, Leeka Bombs. Within
a few months Georgie and Leeka had enjoyed a HolidayDeck
wedding and established a HolidayDeck love nest. But when

Leeka announced that she was in a HolidayDeck family way, Georgie panicked and ended the program.

Capt. Ricardo and his brother Rodney Ricardo had been the toast of the all-star mud-wrestling and wine-tasting circuit in France for awhile. Then the grapes had an off year, public interest in mud wrestling waned, the circuit closed down, and the wrasslin' Ricardos were out of work.

And so all of Ricardo's crewmembers had drifted back to Starfreak Headquarters within the last month or so. However, Starfreak Command, nursing a grudge over the crew's role in losing the Fountain of Youth to the Romanumens, hadn't been in any hurry to give them a new mission.

The crew also knew that their permanent status was in jeopardy because their agreement with Starfreak expired when the last of the fountain water was gone. So they'd reluctantly agreed to attend this seminar on political correctness to get on the good side of Starfreak Command.

That is, most of them came reluctantly. Capt. Ricardo was the exception—he thought it was a jolly good idea. Now he was taking notes as the speaker outlined the day's program.

"During our breakout sessions," the speaker said, "you'll learn the correct attitudes toward multi-sexual beings, aliens of color, disenfranchised life forms, and other groups. You'll discover why your present approach to your Starfreak duties is sexist, racist, ageist, and sentientist. By the end of this seminar, you'll be groveling for forgiveness to alien beings that you aren't even aware of right now, and admitting that you are the scum of the galaxy. Okay, everybody ready? Let's get started!"

Capt. Ricardo felt pretty smug at the beginning of his first breakout session, an encounter group for starship captains. Ricardo studied his peers and guessed that he was as politically correct as any of them. As they went around the circle and introduced themselves, he scored a few points by apologizing for being a white male.

Then it came time to focus more intensely on each individual's track record. Ricardo's name happened to come up first, and the others began questioning him.

"Captain Ricardo, what's your stand on opportunities for women?" one captain inquired.

"I'm glad you asked," Ricardo replied, smiling with as much sincerity as he could muster. "My crew includes women in a number of important positions."

"Which positions?" she pressed.

"My chief medical officer is female, as is my ship's counselor," Ricardo answered.

"Hmmph," somebody sniffed, "medicine and counseling. The traditional female 'helping' professions. Anybody else?"

"Uh, well," said Ricardo, momentarily taken aback, "there is Guano."

"And what does this 'Guano' do?" the first woman asked.

"She's, er, she's the head bartender in our Ten-Foreplay lounge," Ricardo responded.

"The head bartender?" someone else echoed.

"And a very important position it is, too," Ricardo maintained stoutly. "She's a good listener, and she often provides a shoulder to cry on or gives a bit of good advice to a confused crewmember."

"Isn't that the responsibility of your ship's counselor?" asked another captain.

"Well, er, yes," Ricardo stumbled, "these are things that Counselor Troit does, but Guano also does them for crewmembers in Ten-Foreplay, when, ah, when they're...."

"Drunk?" someone else supplied.

"Captain Ricardo," said the group leader, "according to the questionnaire you filled out for this seminar, your Bridge crew doesn't contain any Hispanics or Asians. Would you mind explaining why?"

"Well, I, uh ... it's certainly not intentional ... " Ricardo stuttered. "I suppose I've never looked at it that way."

"Just how many minorities are there on your Bridge crew, Captain Ricardo?"

"There's Wart, my security officer," Ricardo said. "He is a Kringle—"

"An aggressive, warlike race that hardly qualifies as an oppressed minority," someone stated.

"And then there's Lieutenant Commander Dacron, an android," Ricardo said, pulling nervously at his collar. "Very few starships have an android among their senior officers, you know."

"So what?" another captain challenged. "He's a male, isn't he?"

"Yes, he is," Ricardo said.

"Does he have any redeeming color value? Is he purple, magenta, polka-dotted? Anything highly unusual?"

"Not really," said Ricardo.

"Just what color is he, Captain?"

Capt. Ricardo swallowed hard and admitted, "White. Dacron is extremely white." A chill of disapproval swept through the group.

Another captain broke in. "Captain Ricardo, what about equal opportunities for animals?"

Ricardo crossed his legs and jiggled his foot nervously. "Animals . . . animals . . . let's see . . . " he said. "Ah, yes. One of my senior officers has a pet named Spot."

"Oh, so you do provide opportunities for dogs, then?"

"Er, no," Ricardo said, jiggling his foot a little faster. "We don't have any dogs. Actually, Spot is a cat." He grinned broadly at the group; cold stares answered him. His grin wilted as he attempted to explain: "Since this was the first pet among the senior officers, and Spot is a traditional pet name, Dacron thought it would be amusing to give it that name, despite the fact that it's a cat, not a dog—"

"This Dacron, who gave the cat its name," somebody interrupted, "is he the albino android?"

"He's not an albino," Ricardo replied testily. "He—"

Mercifully, at that moment the intercom interrupted them. "Captain Ricardo, this is Admiral Less," came the voice. "Report to my office at once."

Ricardo stood up and began backing out of the room. "So sorry to have to end this line of questioning," he said, facing down the others' glares. "It's really been quite . . . quite . . . enlightening." Then he turned and darted out the door before anyone could ask another question.

As he headed down the hall, wiping perspiration from his brow, Ricardo wondered what kind of score the others would give him on their evaluation sheets. At least no one had thought to ask about the race and sex of his first officer.

"Sit down, Captain, and relax. I won't bite," said Admiral Less with a hint of a sly grin. She was obviously enjoying Ricardo's discomfort.

It wasn't the possibility of getting bitten that Ricardo was worried about; it was the chance of being stabbed by that menacing fingernail of hers. He tried to relax, but the horsehair guest chair made him fidget, as it undoubtedly was designed to do.

He had talked to plenty of admirals before, but those conversations usually took place over the Viewscreen as he stood in the comfort of his own Bridge. Being here on Starfreak territory was considerably more intimidating.

"Starfreak has a mission for you, Captain," said Admiral Less. "You're familiar with the recent actions of Captain James T. Smirk and his crew—the way they refused the order to retire and then commandeered their ship?"

Ricardo nodded. Indeed, he'd followed the story more closely than most. Mandatory retirement weighed heavily on his mind these days, and he secretly wondered if he too would have the courage to resist being put out to pasture when his own time came.

"Obviously, Starfreak cannot let this action go unchallenged," Less went on. "But now there's much more to it than that. I'll let this videotape explain."

Admiral Less popped the tape into her desktop VCR, and they turned to watch her portable Viewscreen. The image that appeared there was a little shaky—the tape had obviously been made with a handheld camera—but the subject was unmistakable: it was Capt. Smirk. He was standing in the middle of an outdoor fountain, gaily splashing water with his hands.

"Starfreak Command, this is Captain Smirk!" he said to the camera. "I thought you'd like to know that my crew has driven the Romanumens off this planet and claimed the Fountain of Youth. Perhaps we could negotiate a reinstatement of my crew in return for my sending a portion of the fountain's water to Starfreak. So what do you say? Do we have a deal?"

A water pistol appeared in the foreground, and someone began firing it at Capt. Smirk. "Checkout, knock it off!" Smirk protested cheerfully. He splashed water in Checkout's direction; a few drops beaded up on the camera lens. "I'll be waiting to hear from you, Starfreak!" Smirk concluded, signing off with the two-fingered peace sign.

Admiral Less switched off the VCR and told Ricardo, "Our intelligence reports confirm what Smirk said. He did drive the Romanumens off the planet. Don't ask me how, with one starship and a tiny, over-the-hill crew. Perhaps the Romanumens became complacent after Starfreak officially gave up on the fountain.

"So now we've got a renegade Starfreak officer holding the most valuable asset in that sector. Obviously, Captain Ricardo, your mission is to get it back for us."

Ricardo ventured, "You're not going to bargain with him?"

"Bargain? What for? He had no right to use that starship in the first place," Less maintained. "As a matter of fact, right now there are seven spots at the Vacant Attic Nursing Home awaiting him and his cronies. After you've recovered the Fountain of Youth, you're to deliver Smirk and his crew to the nursing home."

"I see," Ricardo answered. Suddenly the mission took on greater interest for him. Finally, here was a chance for his crew to wreak revenge on their rivals—and with Starfreak's blessing, to boot.

"Of course, this reinstatement of your crew is just a trial

period, Captain," the admiral went on. "But once you carry out the mission, Starfreak will profit from the sale of the Fountain of Youth's water, and some of that money can be earmarked to keep your *Endocrine* in service. Consider yourself lucky—a lot of our other ships are still in the shop for repairs after the Bored War."

"Very good, Admiral," Ricardo said. Already he was aching to get on with the mission. *Look out, Smirk, you cocky jackanapes,* he thought. *This is my crew's chance to make it clear, once and for all, that we're the only* Endocrine.

As Capt. Ricardo's ship made its way toward the planet Smirk had taken over, Ricardo was puttering in his Ready Room when an unexpected visitor arrived.

The visitor couldn't have come at a worse time. Ricardo's right arm was immersed up to the elbow in the built-in fish tank in the corner. He'd removed the cover to check the filter pump, and one of the gold pips on his collar had fallen into the tank. Now he was trying to retrieve the pip before the expensive kissing gouramis might try to swallow it and kill themselves.

The visitor appeared in a flash of light, startling Ricardo so that he dropped the net he was using to retrieve the pip. "Hello there, *mon Capricorn*," said the intruder.

Ricardo whirled around and snapped at him, "Q-Tip! Don't you ever knock?"

"Why should I?" Q-Tip replied, lounging across Ricardo's desk and fiddling with the pen-and-pencil set. He was in the humanoid form he usually adopted for visits to the *Endocrine*. "As part of a continuum of omnipotent beings, I feel entitled simply to barge in at will. You should be used to that by now." Q-Tip peered at Ricardo. "Whatever are you doing to that poor fish?" he inquired.

Turning his gaze from Q-Tip back to the fish tank, Ricardo realized that he'd snared a fish's fin with his net. "Drat," he muttered, gently shaking the net to try to release the fish;

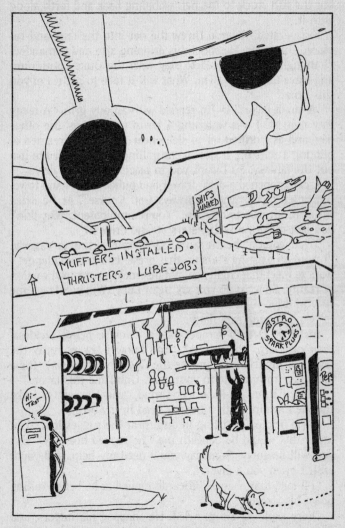

"A lot of our other ships are still in the shop for repairs."

but the fish stuck to the net, wobbling back and forth along with it.

Exasperated, Ricardo threw the net into the tank and replaced the cover. He shook his dripping arm and demanded, "I thought you'd agreed to stay with the Quke continuum and leave us alone, Q-Tip. What will it take to get rid of you this time?"

"A small favor," Q-Tip replied with an oily grin. "A teeny tiny request. I was watching a rerun of 'Cosmos' the other day, and as I drifted off to sleep near the end, I dreamed of piloting a starship. It was so enthralling that I decided to live out the fantasy. So I want you to teach me how to drive."

Ricardo opened a desk drawer and pulled out a hand towel imprinted "Valleywood Fairways Golf Course." As he dried his arm, Ricardo told Q-Tip, "You're omnipotent. Why don't you just make yourself a starship and drive it?"

"That wouldn't be the same," Q-Tip said, sitting up eagerly. "I need an existing starship that presents a real challenge. I want to meet that challenge, not just make up my own version of reality. So what do you say, Jean-Lucy? Will you teach me how to drive your ship?"

"No," Ricardo said flatly.

Instantly Q-Tip's temper flared. "You're being reckless, *mon capillary*," he warned. "You know I always repay the favors of my friends. I'm like the Godfather that way. It's a good idea to have me in your debt. Grant me this favor."

"And if I don't," Ricardo retorted, "can I expect to wake up one morning with a horse's head in my bed?"

Q-Tip bridled, snorting in disgust at the suggestion. "You know that would be beneath me," he replied hoarsely. "But you will be sorry. Someday you'll need my help, and you'll wish I owed you a favor."

"I'll take that chance," Ricardo replied as he began rolling down his sleeve.

"Very well," Q-Tip growled. He snapped his fingers, and Ricardo felt a strange tug at his collar and heard the kissing gouramis splash around in their tank. Then Q-Tip disappeared in a flash of light.

Wondering what Q-Tip had just pulled off, Ricardo strolled over to the corner. A glance at the fish tank and a quick feel of his collar confirmed his suspicion: now all four of his pips lay at the bottom of the tank.

As Q-Tip and Ricardo were chatting in the Ready Room, Dacron was entering the Ten-Foreplay lounge for his afternoon break.

But instead of her usual cheerful greeting, Chief Bartender Guano gave him an eerie stare. Dacron sat on a barstool and inquired, "Is something wrong, Guano?"

"Yes," she replied. "It's you. You're not supposed to be here."

"Oh," said Dacron. He thought for a moment, then pulled out his wallet. "Here is my ID," he offered. "It proves that I have reached legal drinking age."

"No, no, Dacron," said Guano. "It's not that. I mean you're not supposed to be here in this timeline. This is all wrong somehow."

Dacron was puzzled. "I do not understand."

"Neither do I," Guano said, "but I got this same creepy feeling when your old dead crewmate Yasha Tar showed up. Remember? Somehow she'd slipped into the wrong timeline and turned up alive again here on the ship."

Dacron pondered the meaning of this. "Do you think that the same sort of fate is in store for me?" he asked. Both he and Guano knew what had eventually happened to the misplaced Yasha: she'd returned to her proper timeline and got caught in a deadly battle aboard the *Endocrine C-Sick*.

"I don't know," Guano replied in a raspy whisper. She shivered.

Dacron asked, "Do you believe in omens, Guano?" When the chief bartender nodded, Dacron continued, "Yesterday I accidentally dropped a bottle of Tarium-Three on my cat,

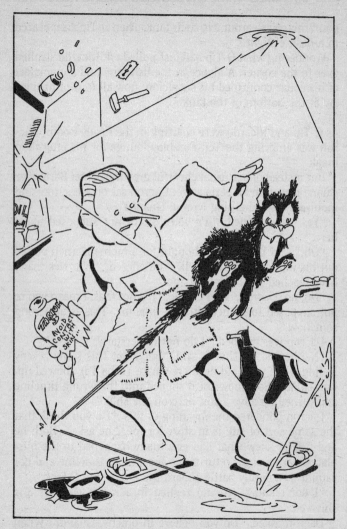

"Yesterday I accidentally dropped a bottle of Tarium-Three on my cat."

Spot, turning him into a black cat. Since then he has crossed my path fifty-seven times."

Guano shuddered. "Have you had any other signs of bad luck lately?" she asked. "Have you broken a mirror or anything?"

"Yes, I have," Dacron answered. "I dropped the main operating mirror while adjusting one of our deflector screens this morning. But I did not realize until this moment that it had significance beyond the fact that it will cost three times my annual salary to replace."

"Oooh. This is bad," moaned Guano. "This is really bad." She shook her head.

Dacron grasped her arm, looking increasingly worried. "What should I do, Guano?" he asked. "What is in store for me?"

"There's only one way to find out," said Guano. She ducked behind the counter for several moments. Dacron leaned over the bar, trying to see what was going on. Soon Guano reappeared wearing a fortune-teller's black gown and a sorcerer's pointy hat. She placed a novelty toy, the 8-Ball, on the counter.

"This is our guide to the spirit world," she told Dacron. "The 8-Ball never lies." Examining the ball, Dacron found a plastic window at its bottom. As he watched, a cube floated into view in the window, reading "Maybe so." He turned the 8-Ball right side up, then upside down, and checked the window again; this time it read "Nevermore."

"This will tell us your fate," Guano stated. "Oh, powerful 8-Ball," she declaimed loudly, drawing stares from other patrons at the bar, "reveal your truth to us. Is Dacron in trouble?" Guano nodded at Dacron; he shook the ball and turned it upside down. The reply read "Yep."

Dacron and Guano looked at each other in alarm. Guano asked, "Oh, 8-Ball, is Dacron in any physical danger?" Dacron shook the 8-Ball an extra long time to make sure it was randomly mixed; then he turned it upside down. An answer floated into view: "Real bad."

Now Dacron and Guano were thoroughly hooked by the mystery.

Now Dacron and Guano were thoroughly hooked by the mystery. Guano, her voice trembling, asked her final question, "Oh, 8-Ball, is Dacron going to die?"

Together Dacron and Guano shook the 8-Ball, round and round and round, till they could delay no longer. They turned the ball over carefully. The answer floated into view:

"You betcha."

By the time Capt. Ricardo's crew arrived at the planet where Capt. Smirk was holding the Fountain of Youth, Ricardo's resolve to smash his rival had withered somewhat. Ricardo stood in the center of his Bridge, studying the planet's surface in the Viewscreen as he silently suffered the slings and arrows of his chronic condition: an overdeveloped conscience.

Smirk is only doing what I would do in the same situation, Ricardo thought. *As a fellow captain, shouldn't I come to his aid instead of doing the dirty work for Starfreak's bureaucracy? He hasn't really done anything this nasty to me. As a matter of fact, he has actually helped us in the past, like when we teamed up to defeat the Cellulites, and when he blew up his ship to destroy the Jargonites.*

Dash it all! Why couldn't he just settle down into a peaceful retirement? Instead he pulls another foolhardy stunt that puts me in the middle.

But if I don't pry him loose from this planet, Starfreak will suspend my crew and then send someone else to do the job. One way or another, Smirk's days are numbered. Might as well get on with it.

"Standard orbit," Ricardo ordered the nameless ensign-of-the-week occupying the Conn station. The ship settled into an orbit of the planet Smirk had captured.

"Mr. Wart," Ricardo continued, "open a channel to the surface."

" 'Hey, you' frequencies open, sir," Wart reported from his Tactical station at the back of the Bridge.

Capt. Smirk appeared on the Viewscreen in dazzling white sports togs. An embroidered "I ♥ tennis" headband propped up the moist curls on his forehead. "Ricardo!" he said with a grin. "Why don't you Fax on down here for a match? I just beat Mr. Zulu in straight sets."

"No, thank you," Ricardo responded with a polite smile. "We're here on an official mission, Captain Smirk. I'm afraid we must take you and your crew into custody and transport you to the Vacant Attic Nursing Home."

"Oh, c'mon, Jean-Lucy. You can't be serious," Smirk responded. "Do I look like someone who's ready to be put out to pasture?"

Ricardo squinted at the Viewscreen. Smirk's face *did* have fewer creases than Ricardo remembered, and Smirk seemed to be bursting with energy. He even appeared to be sporting real hair, not that tacky hairpiece he'd taken to wearing lately.

Ricardo shook his head to ward off the confusion of these new developments. "That's irrelevant," he told Smirk. "My orders are to claim this planet for Starfreak. And you, Captain, have violated a direct order from an admiral. I have no choice but to arrest you."

"Of course you have a choice," Smirk said, deftly flipping off the headband and wringing the sweat from it. "You and your crew could join me down here. With both of our ships guarding the planet, we'd be invincible against any further assaults that Starfreak might send. We'll spend our days playing in the fountain, and our nights living it up. What d'ya say, Jean-Lucy?"

Smirk's offer was so tempting that for a moment Capt. Ricardo wobbled on the edge of uncertainty. Then his conscience began to throb, and he became himself again.

"Certainly not," he said icily. He turned toward the Oops station and ordered, "Mr. Dacron, inform Shipping and Receiving to lock on to Captain Smirk's crew and UltraFax them to our Maximum Security Guest Quarters."

"I wouldn't do that if I were you," Smirk warned them in a lilting singsong.

Dacron consulted his console and reported, "Shipping is ready to transport, sir."

Ricardo, hands on his hips, settled his face into an intimidating stare worthy of Clint Eastwood and ordered, "Go ahead. Make it so."

Moments after the UltraFax beam was activated, an explosion shook the ship. Capt. Ricardo, teetering to recover his balance, ordered, "Damage report!"

"Captain," came Georgie's voice over the intercom from Engineering, "there's some kind of force field protecting the entire planet. Its energy source is Captain Smirk's ship, which is parked in the northeast quadrant. The field bounced our UltraFax beam back to us and damaged our shields. There's a hole in the main shield array. I'm going to have to climb out there with my patch kit to fix it."

"Captain," Wart broke in, "I recommend we fire a full array of futon torpedoes to break the planet's protective field."

"I disagree," Georgie's voice continued. "The futons could boomerang back to us, too. In fact, any weapon we use would bounce right back and hurt us instead of them. This is no ordinary force field. I've seen this before. It's a Colgate Invisible Shield."

"Understood," Capt. Ricardo said to the intercom. He continued, "Mr. Wart, power down all weapons systems."

Bitterly disappointed, as he always was when he didn't get to fire a weapon, Wart did as ordered, then vented his frustration by kicking a hole in one of the science station cabinets at the back of the Bridge.

Ricardo, returning his attention to the Viewscreen, saw that Smirk was making eyes at Counselor Troit, who sat at her regular Bridge station. "Captain Smirk, do you mind?" Ricardo interrupted loudly. Troit blushed and looked away. Smirk turned toward Ricardo with a grin.

"It's been nice seeing you all again," Smirk said. "Some more than others," he added with a significant glance at Troit. "But I've got to go now. I've got an appointment with my personal trainer in the Nautilus room in ten minutes. See you." Abruptly he flicked off his transmission to the Viewscreen.

"But—" Capt. Ricardo started to protest; then he went slack with resignation. He realized he'd never outtalk his rival. But the encounter had given him an idea on how they could get a foothold with Smirk.

"Counselor Troit," he said, turning toward her, "see me in my Ready Room immediately."

"Don't think of it as treachery," Ricardo told Troit a few minutes later, as she started to object to the orders he'd just given her. Ricardo folded his hands, leaned forward on his Ready Room desk, and continued, "Think of yourself as the Mata Hari of Starfreak."

"But sir," Troit protested, "you're asking me to trade on my personal relationship with Captain Smirk just to gain his confidence and gather intelligence about what's going on down there."

"Well . . . yes," said Ricardo. "I didn't expect you to object, Counselor. I thought you'd given up any romantic interest in Captain Smirk long ago, when you broke off your engagement to him and accompanied Dacron to Milwaukee."

Troit wrinkled her face with chagrin. "It's amazing what a few months with an android did to my perspective," she mused, "especially after Dacron's metabolism ran out of Fountain of Love water. It was like living with the Encyclopedia Britannica."

"All right, so Smirk looks more like the last of the red hot lovers than ever," Ricardo acknowledged, trying to stifle his growing irritation. *Why do so many of my crewmembers fight my wishes?* he wondered. *It's such a bother when they have a mind of their own. Why can't more of them be like Commander Piker—brain dead?*

He continued, "Regardless of your personal feelings, Deanna, you've got to help us succeed in this mission. If we don't, Starfreak will fire us again. And they'll send someone else to take Smirk into custody. Either way, he's going to have to face his retirement. So why not do what you can to make the transition as painless as possible? Maybe you can even talk him into surrendering."

Troit sighed. "I suppose so," she agreed.

"Good," Ricardo said with finality. "You may contact Captain Smirk on your personal Viewscreen. Get him to lift this force field long enough for you to UltraFax down. Once you're there, try to find out about this force field or anything else that might help us."

Once the shock of the 8-Ball's dire prediction had worn off a little, Dacron decided to seek a second opinion. Guano agreed that it would be wise to get another, more rational perspective on the issue, so she offered the use of her Ouija Board.

She set the board on the bar, and Dacron sat on a barstool facing her. Together they rested their fingertips on the planchette.

The Ouija quickly confirmed the 8-Ball's prediction that Dacron was going to die. It also hinted that Dacron's death would be slow and painful, triggered by a freak occurrence that would unfold into dire consequences somewhere down the line.

Recalling Yasha Tar's demise, Dacron asked, "Mr. Ouija, will my death occur in the line of duty?"

The planchette dragged itself across the board, slowly spelling out its reply: "SORTA."

Then, remembering the crew's greatest regret at Yasha's death, Dacron asked, "Will it be a senseless death? One which will not further our mission in any way?"

The planchette crept from letter to letter and answered: "TOTALLY SENSELESS."

Dacron was clearly disturbed. "Mr. Ouija," he asked, "can you describe the event that will trigger my death?"

The planchette hesitated in the middle of the board for nearly a minute. Then it crept to the side—slowly at first, but soon picking up speed. Dacron and Guano shifted position to keep their fingertips resting on the planchette as it ran off the board. To their amazement, the planchette slid across the surface of the bar and dropped off the edge.

"Oh, brother," Guano griped as Dacron bent to retrieve it. "This board must need repair." Dacron put the planchette back on the board, and the two placed their hands on it again. "All right, Ouija, I want a straight answer," Guano chided. "Now will you please describe the event that will trigger Dacron's death?"

The planchette began sliding from one letter to another, much faster this time, and with a definite edge to its movements as if the board were angry at them. The reply came: "THAT WAS THE ANSWER YOU IDIOT." Again the planchette slid off the board, skidded across the bar, and plunged to the floor.

3

You're Not Getting Older, You're Getting Younger

CAPT. RICARDO AWOKE with a start and looked around, wondering, *Where am I*? Then he relaxed as he realized he was on the Bridge and had simply fallen asleep again. *They make these chairs too darned comfortable*, he rationalized.

Ricardo pulled the side lever to lower the footrest on his La-Z-Boy command chair. Standing up, he faltered momentarily; his left leg had fallen asleep.

Instantly Piker leaped up and steadied him by the elbow. "Are you all right, sir?" he inquired.

"I'm fine, Number 1," Ricardo assured him. "Just a bit of a cramp in my calf."

"Of course, sir." Piker flashed the fawning grin characteristic of first officers and vice presidents throughout the galaxy.

Ricardo limped over to Dacron's Oops station at the forward section of the Bridge. "How long has Counselor Troit been down on the planet, Dacron?" he asked.

"Exactly thirty-two hours, nine minutes and six seconds, sir," Dacron replied.

"And there's been no change in the sensor readings?" Ricardo pressed. "No break in the Colgate force field? No way to lock on to her signal from here?"

"That is correct, sir," Dacron said. "We have no way of tracking Counselor Troit, nor of retrieving her with our UltraFax beam, until Captain Smirk allows her to make contact." Then a light flashed on Dacron's console. "Captain," he continued, "sensors show a slight break in the force field. It lasted three-point-two seconds and was accompanied by UltraFax beam activity."

Capt. Ricardo hailed Shipping and Receiving via the intercom and confirmed what he'd hoped: Counselor Troit had just Faxed back onto the ship. He instructed her to report to his Ready Room at once.

Capt. Ricardo studied Counselor Troit as she sat down in one of the chairs facing his Ready Room desk. From the look on her face, he guessed that she'd made significant progress with Capt. Smirk. Ricardo noted that Troit's eager, excited expression actually transformed her features so much that she looked years younger.

"Counselor," Ricardo began, "was your mission a success?"

"Oh yeah!" she bubbled. "It's, like, *so* cool down there, you know? I could have just stayed forever."

Ricardo smiled politely. "I'm sure it's a very nice planet," he assented. "Were you able to find out anything about how we can break this force field?"

"Well, no," she admitted. "But, you know, there just wasn't any chance to ask about it without being too pushy. I mean, here I am, UltraFaxing down, and Captain Smirk is like, hey, baby, it's so good to see you again, and I'm like, yeah, I'm glad to see you too, and he's like, do you wanna see the buildings we put up here, and I'm like, sure, let's go. So it would have been pretty phony to break in and go, so, hey, tell me all about this force field around your planet! You know?"

Ricardo stared at her. "Deanna, are you feeling all right?"

"I'm fine," she answered breezily. She fingered a lock of her long hair, holding it up to the light to inspect it for split ends. "Why?"

"You don't sound like your usual self," Ricardo told her.

"I'm just so excited after seeing Captain Smirk again," Deanna revealed. She pulled out a pack of gum and held it toward Capt. Ricardo. "Want some?" He shook his head. She unwrapped a stick of gum and crammed it into her mouth.

"I'm not sure what he's up to," Deanna continued, chomping the gum vigorously, "but there's a lot of stuff going on down there. He invited me to come back whenever I want. Maybe I should go back down there right now, huh? This time maybe he'll tell me about this force field thing you wanted to know." She bounced up out of her chair. "Okay?"

Capt. Ricardo, at a loss for words, simply nodded in agreement. Together they headed out of the Ready Room.

Troit flitted around the Bridge from one crewmember to another. "Guess what, guys?" she squeaked. "I'm going back down to the planet." She squeezed Dacron's shoulder, and he gave her a bewildered look. "Gonna spend more time with this real hunky captain," she went on, skipping over to Piker and ruffling his hair with her hand. She plopped into the captain's chair for a moment and swung her legs with abandon. Then she jumped up again and skipped toward the Crewmover. "This is gonna be *so* great!" she exclaimed. As the Crewmover doors closed, she waved and called, " 'Bye now! Catch ya later!"

Piker smoothed his hair back into place and, as Ricardo settled into the captain's chair to his left, Piker demanded, "What's with her?"

"I'm not sure," Ricardo said. He wasn't sure why Deanna was carrying on so. He wasn't sure she'd be able to gather the information they needed. He wasn't even sure she'd manage to avoid another dangerous infatuation with the smooth-talking Smirk.

Ricardo grimaced. He was only sure of one thing: Deanna had discarded her gum by sticking it onto his chair cushion—and he'd just sat in it.

That afternoon, Dacron spent his off-duty hours in his quarters putting his affairs in order, since no less an authority than Guano's 8-Ball and Ouija Board had both decreed he was going to die.

First Dacron made sure his insurance premiums were paid. Then he set up a trust fund ensuring that Spot would be well cared for. Finally, he sorted through his possessions and discarded those that might cause him post-mortem embarrassment if viewed by others, such as the videotape he and Yasha Tar had made long ago during their brief but torrid tryst.

When all the details were taken care of, Dacron paused, unsure what to do next and wondering how to tell whether death was imminent. He decided to lie down and wait for the Great Spirit to overtake him. Stretching himself out on the bed and lying on his back, Dacron declared aloud, "It is a good day to die."

Within a few minutes, Dacron drifted into a state of deep meditation. Spot ambled into the room, nosed around the edge of the mattress for a moment, then jumped onto Dacron's stomach. Startled, Dacron doubled up, wrenching his back. Spot hissed at him and ran away.

Massaging his aching android muscles, Dacron hobbled over to his medicine chest for some Doan's Pills. He concluded that perhaps his time had not yet come, after all.

It was suppertime, and Smartalecsander sat at the dining table in Wart's quarters staring at his plate. Wart admonished his son, "Eat your supper, young man."

"I don't wanna eat it," Smartalecsander whined. "Why do I hafta eat this baby food? I want to eat what you're eating."

"Traditional Kringle fare is too rich for a youngster," Wart told him. His own plate held a goulash of farm-fresh garnishktz intestines and markklomm sinew.

"It's not fair," moped Smartalecsander. "My food isn't even moving." He plopped his spoon up and down in his mashed potatoes.

"Stop that," Wart ordered. Although he sympathized with the boy, he tried his fatherly best to sound stern. "I'm sure there are human children," he began, then hesitated, ". . . somewhere . . . who would be happy to eat what is on your plate. Now eat it!"

For a while, the two of them chewed away in angry silence. Finally Wart made a stab at pleasant dinner conversation. He'd felt a little out of touch with his son's life ever since re-enrolling him in the *Endocrine*'s educational program. "What did you learn in school today, Smartalecsander?" he inquired.

"A buncha stuff about getting along with other people," the boy replied.

"Oh?" Wart asked suspiciously.

"Like how we should all live in peace and harmony," Smartalecsander droned, obviously bored by the lesson, "and how we can work out our differences without resorting to violence. And why people who start wars are bad guys."

"WHAT?!" Wart bellowed, pounding the table so hard that the leech shaker tipped over.

Smartalecsander, alarmed by the outburst, explained meekly, "The teacher said it's better to compromise and live peaceably than to start a war over foolish pride."

"Of all the . . . " Choked with rage, Wart stood up and paced the room several times. He returned to the table and, in a voice tense from his effort at self-control, asked his son, "Did this teacher also present the other side of the argument—why the honor of one's people is important enough to wage war over, even if it means killing every last one of those people?"

"No, Father," Smartalecsander said.

Wart shook his head in disgust. "This is too much," he spat out. "I cannot have you subjected to such propaganda."

Smartalecsander brightened. "You mean I don't hafta go to school anymore?"

"No," Wart answered as a plan formed in his head. Briefly he recalled his doctor's admonition that spending more than a few hours a day with his son could bring on another nervous breakdown. Then he dismissed the thought—this matter was too important to let his own health considerations stand in the way.

"I will teach you myself, Smartalecsander, in the proper Kringle tradition. We will begin your lessons tomorrow."

Wart sat down again and spread his napkin across his lap. "Now eat your green beans," he told the boy, "or you won't get any krshtloff brains for dessert."

"Huh? Wha—what is it?" Capt. Ricardo sat up in bed, his heart pounding from the shock of being awakened by the intercom.

"I am sorry to disturb you, sir," came Dacron's voice over the intercom, "but you asked to be notified immediately when Counselor Troit returned to the ship. She has just Faxed aboard."

"Unnh," Ricardo grunted. "What time is it?" Groping in the dark for the bedside lamp, he knocked down the plastic pan in which his partial had been soaking.

"It is 0300 hours, sir," Dacron replied.

"0300? Uggh—three A.M.," Ricardo groaned. He kicked at his electric blanket and pulled off his nightcap, muttering, "I wish she had the sense to get in at a decent hour."

"Pardon me, sir?" Dacron inquired.

"I wasn't talking to you, Dacron," Ricardo said. "Our conversation is over. The intercom is supposed to sense that."

"The intercom's automatic end-of-conversation sensor has been malfunctioning," Dacron told him. "Georgie will fix it as soon as he receives the parts that are on back order. Until then, we must use an audio code phrase to end all intercom conversations. Over and out."

Capt. Ricardo asked Cmdr. Piker to sit in on this debriefing of Counselor Troit. Ricardo figured that if Troit was as spacey as she'd been the last time, Piker might be able to make some sense of her report; she seemed to be on his wavelength.

Troit flounced into the Ready Room where Ricardo and Piker were already seated. She took the chair next to Piker, flashed him a brilliant smile and said, "Hiya, Will."

"Hello, Deanna," Piker replied, obviously flattered by her momentary attention.

"Counselor Troit," Ricardo began, yawning, "on any future

away missions, I'd appreciate it if you would return at a decent hour so we don't have to hold the debriefing in the middle of the night like this."

Troit pouted. "What's the big deal? I got here as soon as I could." She twisted one of her shoulder-length curls around her finger and fidgeted in the chair. "Are you giving me some kind of curfew or something?"

Capt. Ricardo sighed. "Never mind. We need your report to shed some light on what Captain Smirk is up to. We've observed a number of construction vehicles going to and from the planet."

"We've seen cement-mixer spacecraft," Piker elaborated, "shuttles carrying concrete blocks, and even a landscape-architect craft full of ficus trees. It looks like Smirk is building something down there. What's going on?"

Troit shrugged. "I dunno. I wasn't outside very long this time. Captain Smirk and I spent most of our time in his b— uh, in his living quarters."

Piker seemed not to notice her slip. He went on, "Dacron monitored the force field around the planet. He said it opens up somehow to let these construction vehicles enter, but we haven't figured out how to use the opening to gain access ourselves. Did Smirk say anything about how to enter or leave the force field?"

"Nope," Troit said, studying her fingernails. "We didn't talk about construction vehicles or force fields or any other boring stuff. We had, like, these really meaningful conversations, you know? The kind where you really bare your soul? It was so . . . so . . . real."

A 30-watt light bulb went on inside Piker's head as he realized Deanna was once again romantically interested in Smirk. Jealousy flared as the embers of Piker's long-buried passion for Deanna rekindled, warming his pancreas.

Once, long ago, he and Deanna had been a hot item. At the last second they'd backed away from what would have been a mixed marriage—she had a brain, he didn't. Knowing the odds were stacked against their relationship, they'd decided to break up; but every so often, the vision of "what could have been" would flood them with tenderness and mutual respect.

"So you wasted all your time down there just letting that greaseball sweet-talk you again?" Piker snapped.

"He's not a greaseball," Troit retorted. "You haven't seen him lately. He's, like, so cute. His hair is all thick and fluffy. Anyway, you should talk. You're the one who goes through Alberto VO-5 by the case."

"Stop it, you two," Ricardo interjected. "Counselor, did you—"

Dacron's voice came through over the intercom. "Captain," Dacron said, "Admiral Less is on the main Viewscreen here on the Bridge. She wishes to speak to you immediately."

"I'll be there in a minute, Dacron," Ricardo replied. He grumbled to Piker, "What wonderful timing. We haven't made any headway, and now that witch is going to ask me for a progress report."

"I heard that, Ricardo," crackled Admiral Less' voice over the intercom.

Ricardo winced, suddenly remembering the broken sensor of the intercom. "My apologies, Admiral," he said. "Over and out."

Ricardo turned to Troit. "Counselor, it's obvious you're not yourself lately," he said. "I want you to report to Sick Bay for a checkup by Dr. Flusher."

"But I'm not sick," Troit protested.

"And I want Commander Piker to escort you, to make sure you get there," Ricardo continued. Piker nodded, clasping Troit's forearm.

"All right, I'll go," Troit whined. "Why are you picking on me all of a sudden?"

Piker stood up, gently but firmly pulling Troit with him. "You know, these May–December romances never work out," he told her unsubtly as they approached the door.

"Buzz off," Troit replied. "You don't know Jim like I do.

He's always been young at heart. Not like some stuffy first officers I know."

"Oh, so now Captain Smirk is 'Jim' again, huh?" Piker said.

Their voices faded as they headed for the Crewmover. Capt. Ricardo followed them out of the Ready Room, trudged to the center of the Bridge, and faced the Viewscreen.

Admiral Less' image appeared there in all its nasty glory. It looked as if she'd been tapping her fingernails impatiently on her desk for quite some time; there was a small groove worn into the wood.

"Admiral," Ricardo began as pleasantly as he could, "what keeps you up at this hour?"

"I'm always up, Ricardo," she said. "A long time ago I faced a choice: coffee or sleep. I chose coffee. At sixteen cups a day, sleep becomes irrelevant.

"But let's get down to business," she continued. "What were you saying about not making headway? Haven't you captured the Fountain of Youth yet?"

"No, Admiral," said Ricardo. "We're still trying to find a way to penetrate the force field Captain Smirk has placed around the planet."

"You mean you haven't even been down to the surface?" Admiral Less shrieked.

Sitting at his Oops station, Dacron flinched. His ears were sensitive to high frequencies, and Admiral Less' voice was capable of reaching the dog-whistle range.

"No, we haven't," Ricardo admitted. "But we do have an opening. My ship's counselor, Deanna Troit, has been able to—"

"Don't bore me with the details, Ricardo," Less scolded. Her voice pitch rose further. "Only one thing is important here—results." Dacron reached into his console drawer for a couple of plugs of cotton and tried to stuff them into his ears without drawing attention to himself.

Less went on, "I'm giving you one more chance to arrest Smirk's crew and claim that fountain. If you can't handle the assignment, I'll send in someone else to do it." Her tone became ever more strident and piercing; Dacron winced in pain despite the cotton plugs.

"And if you fail, that's the end of your crew's chance at permanent reinstatement in Starfreak," Less concluded on an excruciatingly high note. Dacron, unable to stand it any longer, covered his ears with his hands and ran shrieking from the Bridge.

Admiral Less observed him from the Viewscreen and remarked, "Well! I'm glad to see that at least one of your officers realizes the gravity of the situation."

Later, after breakfast, Capt. Ricardo walked down the hall to Sick Bay to question Dr. Flusher about Counselor Troit's condition.

On the way there he happened to pass Wart's quarters. A crudely lettered sign was taped to the door: KRINGLE MILITARY ACADEMY / HOME SCHOOLING OUR SPECIALTY. A Kringle military anthem was playing within. Ricardo made a mental note to ask Wart about the situation.

Entering Sick Bay, Ricardo saw Dr. Flusher examining Counselor Troit while Piker hovered next to them, looking concerned. Apparently Piker had overcome his irritation with Troit and had shifted into his protective mode.

"If there's anything I can do, anything at all," Piker was saying as Ricardo approached, "just let me know."

"You can move a couple of feet to the left," Flusher told him. "You're standing in my light."

"Oops. Sorry," Piker said.

"Doctor Flusher," said Capt. Ricardo, "have you made a diagnosis yet?"

Flusher nodded. She excused herself from Troit, escorted the captain into her office, and shut the door. "I've never seen anything like it," Flusher exclaimed.

Ricardo took her statement with a grain of salt; Flusher said this about nearly every condition she treated. Ricardo sometimes wondered why every new case seemed such a revelation to her. Had she spent her internship in one of the narrower subspecialties, like Ferengi gynecology?

"Deanna's riboflavin system has somehow been totally reconfigured," Flusher went on. "Her thiamin mononitrate levels are skyrocketing, yet the corresponding sodium ascorbate ratio is exceedingly low. And the heliovectrometer ratings are off the charts."

Capt. Ricardo blinked; this was all too much to absorb during a morning that had begun at three A.M. "Doctor," he implored, "can you tell me in layman's terms what's going on with Counselor Troit?"

"Captain," said Dr. Flusher, speaking slowly and clearly for emphasis, "physically and emotionally, Deanna has reverted to an earlier age. She's now approximately fifteen again."

" . . . The Battle of Warthogshead, the Battle of Nurshrikk, and the Battle of Krawczyk," Smartalecsander recited.

"You forgot the Battle of Grrzzzzzyk," Wart prompted him. "That comes after Nurshrikk."

"Okay," said Smartalecsander. "Is it time for recess yet, Father?"

"I suppose so," Wart allowed. This was only the first day of his son's home schooling, and they were still sorting out the ground rules. Smartalecsander had been an attentive pupil, and Wart decided he deserved a reward. "I have something for you," Wart told the boy.

Smartalecsander watched eagerly as his father opened a desk drawer and pulled out a package. "I got you this toy," Wart said, handing him the box. "It is similar to one that I enjoyed playing with when I was young."

"Oh, boy!" Smartalecsander exclaimed, ripping open the package. "A G.I. Jones doll!" The stiff soldier doll was dressed in battle fatigues.

"This is a *talking* G.I. Jones model," Wart pointed out. "My G.I. Jones was not capable of speech. You are lucky that such technology is in use today. I'm sure he has many statements to make about duty and honor."

There was a string at the doll's back. Smartalecsander pulled it out to its full length, and as the string wound back, the doll spoke. "Have a nice day," it said.

"What?" Wart asked.

Smartalecsander pulled the string again. This time the doll said, "Let's turn our swords into plowshares."

"*What?*" Wart demanded. He grabbed the package that Smartalecsander had tossed aside. For the first time he noticed the small print on the front: NEW! PEACETIME MODEL. With a grunt of disgust, Wart flung down the box.

Smartalecsander pulled the string once more. "Give peace a chance," said the G.I. Jones doll.

Wart snatched G.I. Jones from the boy's hand. "Let me have that!" he growled. "More sentimentalist propaganda! To think some people would sell this to children just to make a profit . . . " He seemed about to toss the doll into the garbage can, but Smartalecsander spoke up.

"Wait, Father," he said. "Why don't we conduct a ritual execution on him, like you did that time with the goldfish that wouldn't obey orders?"

Capt. Ricardo's plans for a staff meeting that afternoon were bitterly dashed, even before the agenda could be mimeographed. He cursed this cruel twist of fate, but there was no getting around it: the two issues he'd intended to discuss at the meeting had suddenly solved themselves.

The mystery of Counselor Troit's retro-aging was cleared up by someone's offhand remark that she must have had contact with the Fountain of Youth during her visit to Smirk's planet.

The other issue was how the rest of the crew could get around the force field and gain access to the planet, as Troit had. Ricardo envisioned an elaborate scheme in which Troit would get Smirk to Fax her down again while an Away Team would somehow secretly tag along. But that point was also mooted when Dacron noticed that the force field had been turned off.

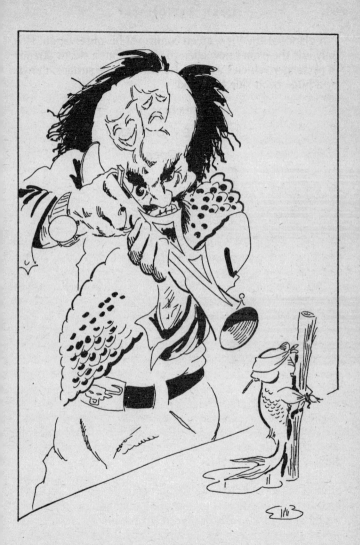

"Why don't we conduct a ritual execution on him?"

A glance at the Viewscreen confirmed his observation. Not only was the planet now open to visitors, but a steady stream of passenger vehicles was headed down to the surface, drawn by a huge neon side that read:

Welcome

JUVEN ISLE THEME PARK

Now Open

4

We Are
Not Amused

THAT SAME DAY, about midmorning, Capt. Ricardo assembled his Away Team in Shipping and Receiving. Now that the force field had been deactivated, they intended to finish their stalled mission: to take Smirk and crew into custody and claim the Fountain of Youth for Starfreak.

Capt. Ricardo was a little nervous about heading into this unknown environment—Juven Isle Theme Park—that Smirk had constructed right under their noses. "Dacron," Ricardo asked, "what did the sensors show about this place?"

"Sensor reports are inconclusive," Dacron replied. "However, I was able to obtain an official guidebook." He opened the guidebook to the page labeled "General Information" and read aloud: "Welcome to Juven Isle Theme Park, designed for the truly young and the youthful wanna-bes. Whether your idea of fun is thrill rides, fast-food stands, musical revues or utterly useless souvenirs, we're here to take your money. All major credit cards are accepted—"

"That's enough, Dacron," Capt. Ricardo broke in. "Apparently Captain Smirk has built himself an amusement park. Since this is Opening Day, he and his crew are probably out on the grounds somewhere. We'll need to locate all of them and bring them back here to the ship. Understood?"

The others nodded. Besides Ricardo, the Away Team consisted of Dacron, Dr. Flusher, and Troit, who was escorted by Piker. Wart was to have come along too, but he begged off at the last minute, citing a conflict between this mission and some kind of father/son social event at Smartalecsander's school. Ricardo made another mental note to ask him what he was up to.

Ricardo stepped onto the UltraFax platform, and the others followed. The Fax beam was set to send them right into the middle of the park. However, in mid-transport, the beam was diverted, and instead they materialized next to the ticket sales booths outside the entrance gate. Unknown to them, an anti-gatecrashers shield protected the park from anyone trying to sneak in via UltraFax without paying admission.

Readjusting their battle plan, they meekly joined the crowds waiting in line to buy tickets. Then, approaching the entrance gate, they faced another challenge. A large sign declared: NO CARRY-IN BOTTLES, CANS, RECORDING EQUIPMENT OR INSIGNIA COMMUNICATORS ALLOWED IN PARK. Reluctantly they surrendered their communicator pins to a security officer. Finally they entered the park itself.

"We'll rendezvous here at 1500 hours," Capt. Ricardo told his crew, pointing to a nearby landmark: a flower bed in which the flowers formed a giant yellow happy face. "Bring with you any members of Captain Smirk's crew you encounter during the day. And stay away from that Fountain of Youth," he warned them. With that, they dispersed to begin the mission.

"Hurry up," Troit urged. "We want to hit the good rides before the lines get too long." She skipped through the crowds clogging the sidewalks, pulling Piker along with her.

"I thought you weren't familiar with what's been going on down here," Piker said, struggling to keep up. "How do you know which rides are good?"

"Jim gave me a sneak preview of some of them," Troit revealed. "I didn't tell Captain Ricardo about it 'cause I was afraid I'd get grounded." Tugging Piker's arm, she added, "Come on, Will. Let's go!"

"Ease up a little, will you?" Piker asked between gulps for air. He wasn't in shape for such an endurance contest, he realized; they must have jogged at least fifty meters already.

"We probably shouldn't be going on any rides, anyway," Piker added. "We're here to capture Smirk's crew, not to have fun."

"Oh, chill out, Will," Troit urged him. "We'll get around to that. Besides, we'll be going on some of the tallest rides. From the top, you'll be able to see the whole park, so it should be pretty easy to spot those guys. Maybe you'll even see them from this first one, the Ferris wheel."

That made sense to Piker. And the gleam in Troit's eye when they reached the Ferocious Ferris gave him another idea: accompanying her on these death-defying thrill rides would definitely be an act of machismo. *She'll probably get scared when we go up high*, Piker thought, *and then I can put my arm around her and make her feel safe. And the thrill of the ride will carry over into how she feels about me. She'll forget all about her crush on Smirk*. The vision was so compelling that it wasn't until they'd waited in line for fifteen minutes and were climbing into the next available seat that Piker remembered he was terrified of heights.

The attendant snapped a metal restraining bar into place across their laps, and the car lurched backward and swayed beneath them. Instantly Piker's sweat glands kicked in; his palms became so slick he could barely grip the bar. He shut his eyes, but that only intensified the sickening feeling as the car swooped up and back.

"Wheeee!" Troit cried. "This is fun!" Piker turned to the side so she wouldn't notice that he couldn't even bear to look.

Finally he realized that if he was going to survey the park for Smirk's crew, he would have to open his eyes while they were at the top, at least for a few seconds. He decided to ease into it by opening his eyes at the bottom first. When the noises and air currents told him they were near the ground, Piker cautiously opened his eyes and looked ahead. They were just passing the lowest point of the wheel's revolution.

Standing on the ground was a young worker in a park maintenance department uniform. Piker shook his head and blinked in astonishment, for the worker seemed to be scraping gum off the underside of the Ferris wheel's seats—while they were in motion. Apparently the park's bubblegum-chewing patrons had wasted no time on Opening Day in marking this new territory, like wolves leaving scent marks around the prairie.

The next time their car reached the bottom, Piker opened his eyes for a longer period and confirmed that the worker was, indeed, trying to clean the cars without stopping the ride. The worker had about five seconds to scrape each car before it swung out of his reach. His timing gradually fell behind, so that after three or four seats had gone by, he got bonked in the back of the head by the next car coming up.

Poor devil, Piker sympathized. *Management probably told him they couldn't afford any downtime while he works on the equipment.*

On the third pass, the young worker's face was visible for a moment, and Piker felt a strange buzz of recognition. It might have been the combination of his dizziness and his impression that this was the ultimate loser's job, but Piker had the fleeting thought that the worker looked just like Checkout would if Checkout were 16 years old.

"Hey, Will, let's rock the car!" Deanna cried, and she began swinging the seat back and forth. Piker's interest in the young maintenance worker vanished as he closed his eyes again and concentrated on not throwing up.

Dacron, wandering among the crowds, soon came up with the same idea that Troit had proposed: the taller rides would provide a good vantage point from which to search for Smirk's crew.

Precise as always, Dacron consulted the guidebook to determine which ride was the tallest. It turned out to be the park's meanest roller coaster, Deathmeister XL-5.

After a long wait in line, Dacron finally boarded one of the cars. A 10-year-old boy plopped into the seat next to him, did a double take upon seeing Dacron's white skin, then cheerily assured Dacron, "Hey, dude, don't be so scared. It's just a ride."

Dacron looked at him in puzzlement for a few seconds; then understanding dawned on his face. "Ah. I see," he said. "You interpret my paleness as an indication of fear over the impending ride. However, that is incorrect. This is my normal skin color."

"Wow. Cool!" the boy exclaimed.

"As a matter of fact, I am looking forward to reaching the tallest peak," Dacron told him.

"You wanna know the best way to ride this ride?" the boy asked as the train of cars lurched forward on the metal track. Dacron nodded. The boy continued, "You've gotta stand up. It's the most awesome feeling."

"But these restraining bars across our laps are designed to prevent such an action," Dacron observed.

"No problem," the boy answered, reaching for a locknut on the lower end of the bar. He gave it a jerk, and the bar swung open. "My friends and I figured this out. We've been on this ride eight times since the park opened this morning." Dacron saw that other youngsters in the cars ahead had loosened their bars, too, and were standing up as the train headed for the first hill.

A sign off to one side ordered REMAIN SEATED, and Dacron noticed that further along in the ride they would be passing through several low tunnels. "Are you certain this is safe?" he inquired.

"I dunno," said the boy. "But it's really fun. Just remember to duck before we hit the tunnels." Dacron hesitated. His seatmate, who was already standing, urged him, "Come on. Don'tcha wanna have fun?"

Dacron looked like he was pondering a foreign concept. "Hmmm. Fun," he mused. "Yes, I believe I do." He stood up, bracing himself as the car ascended the steep angle. A sign at the side of the track read DO NOT STAND. The train clattered up the rails.

Finally the cars reached the top of the first hill and hovered there for an excruciatingly suspenseful moment. Dacron tried to survey the park, but at this height, cirrus clouds blocked their view. Then he looked ahead to where the track took its first plunge down a 78-degree slope.

Instantly Dacron's sensors registered grave danger. His hands locked into a death grip around the restraining bar. The WD-40 chilled in his veins, and his pulse pounded at his temple where an artery fed into his apomecometer.

The cars plunged into a near free-fall. Riders screamed as their primal instincts told them that this was somewhat unnatural. Whomped by G-forces of suffocating intensity, those who'd remained in their seats were plastered against the backrests, and those who were standing clung desperately to the nearest handhold and hung on for their lives.

The cars bottomed out and rushed up the next hill, carrying mighty momentum from their first drop. Then they headed for a series of dips in the track. Some of the dips were covered by the tunnels Dacron had noticed, made from arches of fake rock.

Dacron's seatmate and his buddies sat down, anticipating the low clearance ahead, but Dacron remained standing. In those moments of terror as they'd plunged down the first hill, his hard drive had frozen up, leaving his positronic circuits powerless to evaluate the situation. He stood with his knees locked as the cars approached the tunnel.

"Look out!" yelled the boy, trying to pull Dacron back into his seat, but it was too late. Dacron's head conked against the low arch. Knocked from the car, he fell to the ground some 50 feet below and collapsed in a heap.

As Dacron's hard drive re-booted and he came to his senses, the first thing he saw was a sign propped up against the understructure of the ride. It read: WE TOLD YOU NOT TO STAND.

Gingerly, Dacron examined the spot where the arch had struck his head. His hand came away from his forehead wet with WD-40, so he decided to head for the first-aid station. The guidebook told him it was right next door. *From a liability standpoint, that is probably a good idea*, Dacron reasoned. He tottered over to the station, where a nurse took his name, his temperature, and an imprint of his MasterCard.

Soon after Dacron was seated in one of the treatment rooms, a young medic entered. He took one look at Dacron and exclaimed, "You?!"

"I beg your pardon?" Dacron inquired.

"Uh . . . never mind," the doctor muttered. He seemed to be in a bad mood as he gave Dacron's forehead a cursory examination.

"Please give me the unvarnished truth, Doctor," Dacron requested. "How long do I have to live?"

"Too darned long," mumbled the doctor. "Here, tell me when it hurts." He stuck a knitting-needle-like probe into Dacron's wound.

"Ouch!" Dacron cried.

The doctor withdrew the probe, folded his arms against his chest, and looked down his nose at Dacron. "You park visitors are all the same," the doctor crabbed. "Get a little cut or bruise and you think it's the end of the world. I'm tired of treating these minor injuries. From now on I'm only going to handle wounds that require twenty-five stitches or more, understand? I'm a doctor, not a nurse! Now get out of here. If you're so worried about that itty-bitty cut, go buy a box of Band-Aids at the souvenir stand."

Dacron stumbled out of the first-aid station, trying to figure out what had just happened. The doctor's voice had sounded very much like Dr. McCaw's, yet his young face didn't match up with Dacron's internal file on McCaw. As Dacron's synaptic circuits began to throb, he dismissed the thought and headed for the nearest souvenir stand to buy bandages.

Piker huffed and puffed, trying to keep up with Troit. She was so determined to reach the next "good" ride that they were practically running.

As they rushed through a courtyard on their way across the park, neither of them paid much attention to a strange clown surrounded by a crowd of eager children. The clown's rainbow wig barely concealed his pointy ears. His deadpan expression and sternly slanted eyebrows seemed out of place

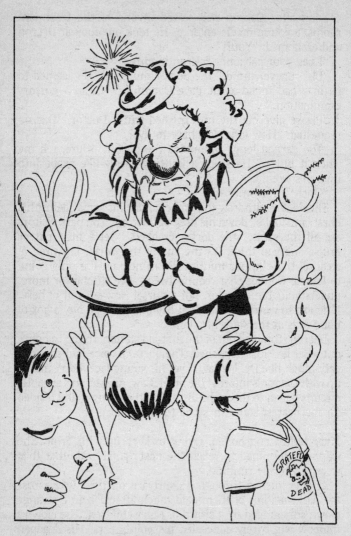

The clown's rainbow wig barely concealed his pointy ears.

as he went about the jolly business of twisting long, thin balloons into animal shapes.

One of the children held up a purple balloon and asked the clown to shape it into a weiner dog. The clown shook his head and told the child, "I am afraid I cannot comply with such an illogical request. Dogs are never purple."

Farther on, Piker and Troit passed the section where the kiddie rides were clustered. Again, they were in too much of a hurry to notice their surroundings. But if they had stopped to investigate, they'd have seen a young Scotsman, his coveralls smeared with grease, who was attempting to repair the Horsey-Go-Round. In his frustration at the balky mechanism, he was screaming so vehemently that parents were covering their children's ears with their hands.

Piker and Troit finally reached their ride and got in line. "This is it," Troit told Piker, rubbing her hands together in anticipation.

They'd arrived at the centerpiece of the park, Juven Isle itself. The island had been constructed of fabricated rock and a jungle of plastic foliage. A moat of water surrounded it, and waterfalls and fountain sprays sprang forth from the rock at various points. Swooping over and under and around it all was a log-flume roller coaster. As the coaster zipped around the island, riders plunged through the water in several places, laughing and shrieking as they became thoroughly soaked.

"This is absolutely the best ride," Troit claimed. "You're gonna love it." She failed to mention that the source of all of Juven Isle's water was the Fountain of Youth. It wasn't labeled as such, but a sign at the entrance gave a clue: DO NOT ATTEMPT TO RIDE THIS ATTRACTION IF YOU SUFFER FROM A HEART CONDITION, ARE PREGNANT, OR DO NOT WANT TO BECOME APPROXIMATELY FIVE YEARS YOUNGER WITH EACH EXPOSURE. Troit giggled mischievously, but Piker, who hadn't noticed the sign, couldn't get her to say why she was so giddy. "You'll see," she said. "Once you ride this ride, you're, like, never the same."

When their turn came, they climbed into a car. Once again,

Piker was too frightened of the height to survey the park as the coaster climbed upward. But after they plunged through the first water drop, which splashed all the riders, he relaxed just a bit.

They got wetter as the coaster whizzed through a bubbly waterfall. *Hey, this is fun*, Piker realized. He laughed with delight, and Troit laughed along with him.

With each plunge, Piker enjoyed the ride more. By the time they passed through the last water trough, where the cars were submerged for a full 15 seconds, he felt exhilarated.

When the ride ended, Troit and Piker ran down the exit ramp to the sidewalk. "That was great!" Piker exclaimed.

"I told you you'd like it," Troit replied.

"What's next?" Piker asked, looking around eagerly. "I'm up for anything!"

The closest thrill ride was the Egg Beater, so they decided to try it. Egg Beater riders were strapped, standing up, onto the spokes of a metal framework. As the ride got underway, the spokes whirled and intertwined faster and faster until they blurred with speed.

Helping people on and then scraping them off this dizzying contraption was a young worker in a park employee's uniform. He was quite helpful, volunteering to hold objects that the riders couldn't take along because they might lose them during the ride—things like stuffed toy prizes, oversized handbags, and false teeth. But what Piker noticed most about him were his strangely familiar Oriental features. Even so, Piker failed to make the connection between this familiar face and his own mission. And as Piker stumbled off the ride, his brain was more scrambled than usual, so he forgot all about the encounter.

Dr. Flusher shifted her weight uneasily from one foot to another and studied the buildings in the park's main courtyard. She was caught in that perennial, unmentionable dilemma of Away Team members: locating the restroom in an alien environment.

Finally she spotted a ladies' room, but her relief was tempered with dismay when she saw that the restroom had a waiting line as long as the lines for any of the amusement rides. In fact, the women were backed up past a sign that said: WAITING TIME FROM THIS POINT—APPROXIMATELY 75 MINUTES.

Finally, after what seemed an eternity, Flusher reached the restroom. Afterward she hobbled out, wondering if her bladder would ever be the same. She didn't feel up to doing much walking, so when she noticed one of the park's theaters, she decided to begin her search there.

Standing up front near the stage, Flusher was able to scan the crowd, but she didn't see anyone from Smirk's crew. Then the house lights dimmed and she was forced to sit down.

An announcer stepped into the spotlight. "Welcome to Broadway Boo-Boos," she said with artificial brightness, "our tribute to a dozen Broadway shows that closed within a week of their opening night. For our first number, from the Broadway adaptation of 'General Hospital,' here's the classic ballad 'Sentimental Gurney'!"

Scattered applause greeted the first singer. With her voluptuous figure and dark-skinned beauty, she made a beautiful first impression. Then she spoiled it by opening her mouth. It sounded as if she was singing in some alien key, one which had several half- and quarter-tones that the human ear couldn't quite assimilate.

I've heard that voice somewhere before, Flusher thought. *I know—it reminds me of Yoohoo rehearsing while we waited to go on stage at that wrekkie convention. But this woman is so young. This can't be Yoohoo ... can it?*

Troit and Piker rode the log flume again. As soon as they got off, they ran back and got in line once more.

When they exited the third time, Piker was whooping with excitement. "That was, like, totally awesome!" he exclaimed in a voice that was much higher than it had been that morning.

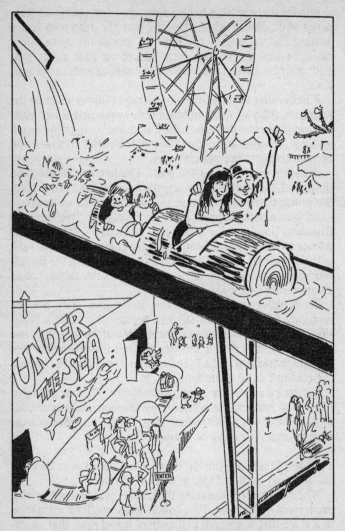

Troit and Piker rode the log flume again.

Troit gave him an adoring glance. The tunic of his uniform hung rather loosely; it looked like he'd shed a lot of weight from his torso. His face was boyish and unlined. The most startling change of all was that his beard had disappeared. His cheeks were now covered with a soft, downy peach-fuzz.

"You were right about these rides, Dee baby," Piker went on. "They're the greatest."

She hugged his waist. "I knew you'd get into this, Will," she replied. "You are just *too* cool."

Suddenly Piker felt certain that he could make Deanna forget all about Smirk. All it took was a little finesse in the romance department, he realized. So Piker hugged Deanna, nuzzled her neck, and gave her an enormous hickey.

5

Death Valley
Days

C APT. RICARDO TOOK a different tack in this search for Smirk's crew than the other Away Team members did. He didn't ride the rides. In fact, he'd never be caught dead on a ride. The whole practice struck him as pointless and undignified. So finding a high vantage point was out of the question.

He didn't visit the musical revues. The last time he'd seen a play was a couple of decades ago, when the musical version of the science fiction classic *Dune* was making the rounds. That had been such a bomb that he'd sworn off theater altogether. So he wasn't about to waste time searching the park's auditoriums.

He didn't visit the souvenir shops. He knew from experience that the clerks would take one look at him and try to sell him a souvenir cap or a bottle of sunblock lotion for his scalp. So if some of Smirk's crewmates happened to be working in the shops, he'd take the chance of missing them.

Instead, Ricardo headed straight for the management office, reasoning that since Smirk was masterminding this project, he had to station himself in a place where he could direct all the action.

Ricardo was right. Approaching the management building, he saw a crowd of teenage girls gathered at the door. At the center of the group stood a handsome young man in baggy surfer shorts and a sweatshirt. Atop his head was a thick cluster of brown curls. They contrasted sharply with the close-shaved sides of his head, into which the initials "JTS" had been carved. He was holding up his hands as if to ward off the females around him.

"Please, please," he said with a smile, "there's only so much of me to go around!"

Capt. Ricardo elbowed his way through the group until he was standing at the young man's side. "Captain Smirk?" Ricardo inquired.

Smirk seemed genuinely happy to see him. "Jean-Lucy," he said, "what's shakin', man?" Ricardo frowned, and Smirk said to the crowd, "Gals, if you'll excuse us for a minute?" The girls sighed with dismay as Smirk escorted Ricardo into the management building and shut the outer door behind them. Ricardo followed Smirk as he headed for an inner office. Its door was plastered with posters of rock bands.

"Have a seat," Smirk invited, sweeping a pile of gym clothes off the guest chair and onto the floor. Ricardo sat down gingerly, as if he feared that relaxing in the chair would make him more susceptible to dirty-clothes germs.

Smirk went around to the other side of the desk, sat in the swivel chair, and put his feet up on the desk. Then he pulled his feet back abruptly and sat up straight. "Sorry to be so rude, man," he said. "Do you want, like, something to drink or something?"

Smirk bounced over to the wet bar behind his desk. He stuck his head inside the small refrigerator, and his voice emerged: "We've got cola, diet cola, orange juice, sports drink, milk, and a pitcher of raspberry Fizzies that I made up this morning."

"No, thank you," Ricardo replied stiffly.

Smirk grabbed a quart of milk, sat in his desk chair again, and swung his feet onto the desk. "I'm glad you made it here on Opening Day," he said. He paused to take a swig of milk from the carton, then continued, "You'll get to see this really boss parade we're having tonight. It'll go down the main promenade." He grinned, and a milk mustache glistened on his upper lip.

"Captain Smirk," Ricardo said, impatient to get on with it, "surely you must know why I'm here."

"You bet your sweet bippy," Smirk replied. "And I can't blame ya. You're gonna see a really groovy change after just one or two trips through the water on Juven Isle. My crew and I practically lived there the first few days after we got here. We were getting so young we had to lay off the water for a while, so we wouldn't turn into babies like the Romanumens did."

"I'm not here for the water," Ricardo snapped. "We've been through all of this already. I'm here to claim the Fountain of Youth for Starfreak and to take you into custody for transport to the nursing home Starfreak has assigned you."

Smirk gazed at Ricardo for a few seconds, then cackled with laughter. Ricardo stared back, flushed with anger. Smirk abandoned himself to his laughter for a minute, then caught his breath and paused to finish off the milk in the carton. After a big swallow, he exclaimed, "Man, you are too much."

Smirk leaned back in his chair and pressed the on/off button of the stereo receiver on the shelf next to his desk. An announcer's voice boomed from the six speakers surrounding the room: "The time is 2:45, and you're listening to WpH1, the home of acid rock."

Smirk crushed the empty milk carton against his desk and tossed it at a wastebasket in the corner that had a small plastic basketball hoop hung over it. The carton sailed neatly through the hoop and into the basket. "Three points!" Smirk exclaimed. Then he turned to Ricardo.

"Sorry to ruin your day, Jean-Lucy, but like I told you before, we're not going," he said. "We've got one terrific operation here. Why should we give it up? Just so Starfreak Command can get a little fatter? No way, man.

"My crew captured this planet fair and square. You think it was fun rounding up all those baby Romanumens into a playpen and then shuttling them to a day-care planet in the next sector? I'm *still* trying to get the spit-up stains out of

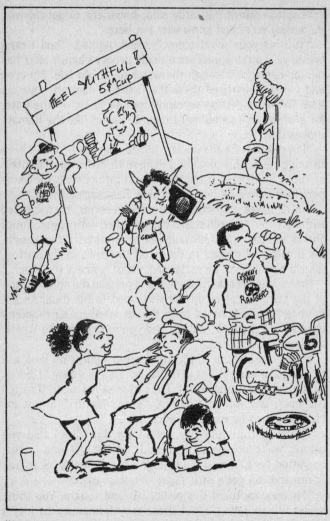

"We were getting so young we had to lay off the water for a while."

my tunic. Yeah, we paid the price to own this fountain, all right. And we're gonna make it pay off."

Smirk paused a moment to groove to the music on the radio broadcast, his upper body swaying to the heavy bass beat as the lead vocalist screamed, *"This must be love, 'cause you make me sweat / It's true love, baby, I'm dripping wet . . ."*

Smirk turned back to their conversation. "Maybe some of my crewmembers aren't crazy about their jobs," he allowed, "but they pitch in 'cause the more profit we make with this park, the more power we have in the federation. It doesn't even matter whether we ever get back in Starfreak. We've got everything we need right here. I don't need to leave my own backyard to meet some of the tastiest chicks in the galaxy. This park attracts hot babes like you wouldn't believe."

"It's unfortunate that you feel you must resist," Ricardo said, his eyes darting nervously back and forth. "But I do have my orders."

"Hey, let's not make a big scene here, okay?" responded Smirk, sensing trouble. "We can all be cool about this."

"Cool?" Ricardo echoed, buying time. He shifted in his chair to distract attention from his hand. In the next instant he reached for his phaser, which was set on "stun."

Smirk's reflexes were sharper than ever. As Ricardo drew the phaser, Smirk lunged for his pneumatic-action super-squirting toy water rifle on the cluttered desktop, took aim, and blasted a spray of frigid water that knocked Ricardo out of his chair. Reaching out to break the fall, Ricardo dropped his phaser.

In an instant Smirk leaped over to Ricardo's side and placed the water rifle at Ricardo's temple. Ricardo lay in a puddle and gazed up at him helplessly, shivering from the icy blast.

"Cool your jets, Jean-Lucy," Smirk suggested. He kicked the phaser out of Ricardo's reach, then extended a hand to help Ricardo to his feet. "Now that you're wet anyway, you might as well go ride the log flume." Ricardo stood up and wrung some of the water out of his tunic.

Smirk put a hand on Ricardo's shoulder, guiding him toward the outer office. "You can stay as long as you wanna here in the park today," Smirk offered. "So can Dacron and Piker and Dr. Flusher," he went on, waving his hand at the far wall, which held a bank of video monitors linked to surveillance cameras set up throughout the park grounds. "And of course Deanna is free to come and go, like, whenever."

They reached the outer door, and Smirk paused. "But, man, don't mess around saying you're gonna take me to some old-fogey nursing home. I mean, do I look like I'm ready to retire?"

Ricardo shook his head.

"Oh-*kay*!" Smirk exclaimed. His mood turned cheery in an instant. He opened the door, and the girls waiting outside started calling his name, squealing, and pushing toward him. Those in the front row clutched at his sweatshirt.

"All right, babes, you win," Smirk cried in mock resignation. "Take me!" With that, he flung himself into the midst of the crowd, prompting a chorus of lustful screams.

By 1500 hours, all the members of the Away Team had straggled back to the happy-face flower bed. After reclaiming their insignia communicators from the park's security office, they Faxed up to their ship.

A few of them took time out to change into dry clothes. Then they convened a meeting in the Conference Room, and Capt. Ricardo briefed them on his encounter with Smirk.

When Ricardo finished his summary, Dr. Flusher spoke up. "So all his crewmembers are younger," she realized. "Then that *was* Yoohoo that I saw in the theater."

"All right, that's two crewmembers accounted for," Ricardo figured. Turning toward Piker, he saw that his first officer was nuzzling Counselor Troit's ear. "Ahem!" Ricardo harrumphed. Troit giggled, and Piker sat up straight, his face reddening.

For the first time since their Away Team had reassembled, Ricardo took a good look at Piker and noticed something significant. Piker looked much younger and thinner—and there was something else different about him, too. "Number 1," Ricardo inquired, "where's your beard?"

Piker shrugged. "I dunno," he said. "I guess I lost it on one of the rides." This struck Troit's funny bone. She held a hand to her mouth to stifle an attack of the giggles, and her shoulders shook as the giggles erupted inward.

Trying to decipher Troit's overreaction, Ricardo peered at her. That raised a new question. "Counselor Troit, what is that on your neck?"

Troit couldn't contain herself any longer. Her laughter burst forth so violently that she had to gasp for air. Instantly Piker caught her mood, and he, too, launched into a laughing fit.

"I see some of us have visited the Fountain of Youth," Dr. Flusher observed. She went to examine the spot that Ricardo had noticed on Troit's neck. After passing her medical tricorder over it, Flusher announced, "It's a Class Four hickey, administered within the past twenty-four hours."

Exasperated at Piker and Troit, Capt. Ricardo decided to continue the debriefing without them while their laughing fit ran its course. Ricardo turned to Dacron and asked, "Mr. Dacron, did you see any members of Captain Smirk's crew while we were down on the planet?"

"No, sir," Dacron replied, holding a hand against his forehead.

"Is something wrong, Dacron?" Ricardo asked.

"It is merely a superficial head wound, Captain," Dacron answered, "one requiring fewer than twenty-five stitches." He paused and seemed to daydream for several seconds. Then he continued with a dazed look, "Nevertheless, bits and bytes have been leaking out of my central processor periodically."

Dr. Flusher left Troit and walked over to Dacron, gently pulled his hand away, and examined the cut. "I'd hardly call this superficial," she judged. "It's a wonder you haven't suffered brain damage, Dacron."

"I have not ruled out the possibility of dain bramage, Doctor," Dacron stated. "I have yet to run a self-diagnostic."

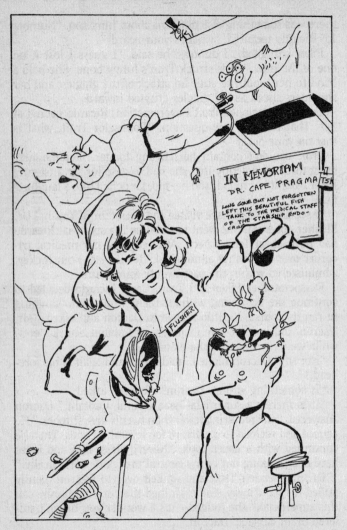

"It's a wonder you haven't suffered brain damage, Dacron."

"We've got to get you to Sick Bay," Flusher ordered, helping him to his feet.

"I would not mind receiving some edical mattention," Dacron admitted. "Perhaps running an anti-virus program would ease this discomfort and clear up my sinuses." His head jerked, his eyes glazed over, and he stated irrelevantly, "Consumes forty-four times its weight in excess stomach acid."

"Please excuse us, Captain," Flusher said as they headed for the door.

Dacron's head jerked again. "Goodbye, all," he said, waving at them awkwardly as he backed out of the room. "Happy trails to you." Flusher pulled him through the doorway.

Piker and Troit finally seemed to be winding down. Sternly Ricardo stared at Troit and asked, "Counselor, you took Commander Piker through the Fountain of Youth, didn't you?"

She nodded. "I hoped it would get him to lighten up," she explained.

Ricardo regretted giving Piker the assignment to keep Troit out of trouble. *Escorting someone whose judgment is impaired is no job for someone who has never had any judgment to begin with*, he realized. *Well, that's all water under the dam now. Or under the flume, as it were.*

Wearily, Ricardo asked, "Did either of you happen to see any of Smirk's crewmates anywhere on the park grounds?"

"No, sir," Piker answered. "But I've got some information that's much more important than that. I wanted you to be the first to know." He put his arm around Troit, squeezed her shoulders, and announced, "Dee and I are going steady."

When the amusement park finally closed late that night, Capt. Smirk's crewmembers returned to their living quarters on Smirk's *Endocrine*, which was parked in the back parking lot.

Although the crew had been young for only a week, they'd already managed to put their mark on the formerly sterile quarters. Clothes were strewn everywhere. Under each bed, a mound of junk included such keepsakes as dirty gym socks, empty cola bottles, magazines, and leftover pizza crusts in cardboard delivery boxes. Visual clutter crept up the walls in the form of posters, souvenirs, crowded bulletin boards and scuff marks from the balls crewmembers tossed around constantly.

Now, as they all returned from their long workday, the living quarters took on the feel of a college dorm. The crewmembers whooped it up, bouncing from one room to another, reliving the day's activities, trashing their rooms to work off nervous energy, and eating whatever they could get their hands on.

Zulu entered McCaw's room and asked him, "Lenny, could I, like, borrow your razor?"

"What for?" taunted McCaw. "You don't shave yet."

"Sure he does," Snot joined in. "He's gonna shave his legs!" He and McCaw burst out laughing. Zulu picked up a pillow and started whacking at their heads.

"Hey, guys," said Capt. Smirk as he entered the room, "did anybody else get a load of the old fogeys' Away Team today?"

"I did," Yoohoo called from across the hall. She sat on her bed painting her toenails, with her toes separated by big fluffy cotton balls. "Dr. Flusher was in the audience watching my noon show, and I'm like, hey, baby, take a lesson from somebody who knows how to *use* it!" Yoohoo wiggled her hips for emphasis, and the others responded with wolf whistles and howls.

"Where did you see them, Captain?" Zulu asked.

"Ricardo comes to my office," Smirk recounted, obviously relishing the tale, "and he goes, so, you guys better come with big bad ol' me, or *else*, and I'm like, give me a break! So he actually pulls out his phaser, that turkey! So I let him have it with the water rifle. Pow!"

Smirk checked his reflection in the mirror over McCaw's dresser and added, "Geez, I wonder if he'll get pneumonia now. They'll hafta put a mustard plaster on his head or something."

"I saw Commander Piker and Counselor Troit riding da

Ferris veel," Checkout offered, slurring his words a little. He was slumped in a chair and holding an ice pack to the egg-sized bump on the back of his head, an occupational injury from being struck by Ferris-wheel seats every 20 seconds. "Piker looked scared. Probably afraid of heights. Vat a chicken." Checkout giggled weakly, then passed out.

"I saw Piker and Troit on my Egg Beater ride," Zulu said. "He looked okay then."

"Speaking of chickens," said McCaw, "that dopey android, Dacron, came in looking for a bandage for his so-called skin. And I'm like, yeah, I've got nothing better to do than hold your hand, yo-yo."

Mr. Smock wasn't there to join the discussion. By midday he'd become fed up with doing balloon tricks for the kiddies, and he'd gone to Capt. Smirk asking for a reassignment. Smirk, admitting that perhaps the clown job didn't make full use of Smock's talents, had decided that Smock should remain on the *Endocrine*'s Bridge and monitor the sensors in case Starfreak had any other sneaky tricks in store for them.

Later that evening, Mr. Smock put the sensors into the "record" mode and joined Zulu, McCaw and Snot as they lounged in McCaw's room, trying to decide how to spend the rest of the night. Capt. Smirk had already left to watch the park's Opening-Night parade along with his dates, four gorgeous gals he'd met that day.

"First we gotta get some real food," Zulu stated. "If I don't get something to eat within fifteen minutes, I'm gonna die."

"Then what?" asked McCaw.

"We could watch TV," Snot suggested. He lay on the bed balancing the remote control channel-changer on his gently rounded tummy. His young fingers had already developed an amazing dexterity at channel-changing.

"There's nothin' on," McCaw told him.

"There's always the Weather Channel," Snot said.

"Nah. That's boring."

"Hey!" Zulu exclaimed. "I know what we can do." He jumped up and shut the door to the outer hallway so Yoohoo wouldn't hear them. "Let's stage a panty raid on Yoohoo's room!"

The others exclaimed: "Yeah!" "Awright!" "Let's do it!"

"Excuse me," Mr. Smock inquired. "What is a panty raid?"

"It's, like, really crazy," Zulu explained, a grin lighting up his face. "You get a buncha guys to charge into some girl's room and go through all their dresser drawers and steal their underpants!"

"And then?" asked Smock, deadpan.

"Well . . . then, that's it," Zulu said, his excitement losing some of its momentum. "You just do it for laughs, you know." Smock's expression reflected his struggle to understand this concept.

"Wait a minute," McCaw said. "Isn't there supposed to be more than one girl? I mean, like, isn't it better if you charge in on where there's a whole buncha girls? Yoohoo probably has only one underwear drawer. We'd have it cleaned out in a few seconds."

"I guess so," Zulu admitted, losing even more enthusiasm. "Well, you got a better idea?"

"There must be somebody we can pick on," Snot said idly, flicking the channel-changer with his forefinger to make it spin round and round on his stomach.

They looked around the room, thinking it over. Eventually, each pair of eyes lit on the same spot: Checkout, slumped in the easy chair, with the now-melted ice bag drooping over his ear.

Sometime around midnight, Checkout awoke. His ice bag was gone. He tried to reach up to feel his injured head, but he couldn't move his arms. Shaking off his stupor, he took a deep breath and realized he was outside in the dark.

He couldn't move his legs, either. He wiggled his fingers, and the scratchy sensation confirmed his worst fear: he'd been buried up to his neck in sand. As his eyes became accustomed to the darkness, he realized he was in the theme park's playground area, smack in the middle of the sandbox.

Checkout sighed deeply and began wriggling his shoulders back and forth, back and forth, half an inch at a time. He knew that although it would be a slow, tedious process, he could eventually dig his way out. He'd done it often enough before.

Midnight marked the end of Admiral Less' normal workday at Starfreak Headquarters. She reached for her lengthy "things to do" list and saw that only one item remained for today: "Reclaim Fountain of Youth for Starfreak."

There had been no further word from Capt. Ricardo, and Less figured this meant he still hadn't made any headway. She decided it was time to send in someone competent to do the job.

She punched a button on her desktop Viewscreen and ordered, "Get me Commander Bungeeman Crisco."

About that same time, on the orbiting *Endocrine*, Capt. Ricardo strolled into Sick Bay. He saw that Dr. Flusher was performing brain surgery on Dacron, who lay on an examination table with his head in a vise. Ricardo turned to leave so he would avoid disturbing Flusher, but she called him back.

"Come in, Captain," she invited. "I can talk to you while I do this. I don't need to concentrate."

Ricardo stepped to the head of the table and observed that Flusher had pried open the top of Dacron's skull. Inside were lots of little blinking lights, whirring gears, and assorted ratchets, rubber-band pulleys, and round Tinker-Toy pieces. "One wonders how it all works," Ricardo marveled.

"Oh, it's pretty straightforward, actually," Flusher told him. With a shiny metal probe, she touched a spot on Dacron's brain; his left leg twitched. She touched another spot, and his right hand jerked; still another, and his Adam's apple bobbed up and down.

"They're all direct connections," Flusher remarked. "In fact, I've dissected frogs with more complex systems than this." She laid the instrument back on the tray, picked up a can of compressed air, and began blowing the dust off Dacron's circuits. "So what brings you here, Captain?"

"I wanted to see whether Dacron would be able to join our Away Team again tomorrow morning," Ricardo said. "And you, too, of course. I'm taking more officers this time. We'll stay in a group, for greater strength."

Flusher nodded, setting aside the can of air spray. She gathered up the used surgical tools from the tray and carried them over to the sink with Ricardo following her. "Dacron should be able to come along," she affirmed. "He may not be up to full speed, but he'll be ambulatory." Turning on the hot-water tap, she squirted some Lemon Fresh Joy over the instruments and began stirring up a froth of bubbles.

"Will Commander Piker and Counselor Troit have come to their senses by then?" Ricardo asked. "I don't want a couple of young whippersnappers on my Away Team," he added with a little grimace of distaste.

"I think so," Flusher said, rinsing the instruments under the faucet and setting them in a plastic utensil holder to dry. "The effects of the fountain's water seem to wear off within twenty-four hours, as long as the person is not re-exposed."

"They won't be," Ricardo told her. "They're under strict orders to stay with the team, and we're not going anywhere near the fountain."

"Then the normal aging process that they'll go through overnight tonight won't be reversed," Flusher affirmed.

The two of them returned to the operating table. Flusher closed the cap on Dacron's skull, released his head from the vise, and reached for the "on" switch on his back. "Okay, Dacron, let's see how you're doing now," she said, flicking the switch.

Nothing happened.

"Hmmmm," said Flusher with the puzzled yet self-assured frown she'd been taught in medical school. She flicked the switch on and off a few times, but Dacron showed no signs of life.

Flusher's expression grew increasingly concerned as she studied the screen of the Scramscope Android Patient Monitor at Dacron's bedside. Apparently she'd somehow failed to notice that sometime within the last few minutes, all of the vital-signs readouts on the screen had gone flat. This meant that either Dacron was dead or someone had tripped over the Scramscope cord again and unplugged it from the wall outlet.

"Nurse Chapstick," Flusher called, "will you get me the Scramscope instruction manual, please?"

"What is it, Doctor?" Ricardo asked, sensing her concern. "You'll be able to revive him, won't you?"

"Of course," Flusher answered, flashing an overly bright smile. "It's just a routine procedure. Meanwhile," she said, steering the captain toward the waiting area of Sick Bay, "why don't you take a seat here and read a few back issues of our in-house publication, *Sick Bay Sentinel*?"

Nervously Ricardo watched from the waiting area as Nurse Chapstick brought Flusher the instruction manual for the monitor. Flusher carefully tested the monitor, double-checked that it was plugged in, and finally, in desperation, gave it a good swift kick. But Dacron's vital signs remained null.

"Code Purple!" Flusher called out. From somewhere in the back of Sick Bay, a team of computer technicians swarmed into the operating area. They re-opened the panel to Dacron's brain and peered inside, using a flashlight to illuminate his mechanism.

After poking around in Dacron's skull for a minute, the chief technician shook his head, and the others solemnly closed the panel. The chief technician said something to Flusher and laid a comforting hand on her shoulder for a moment; then they all filed out the back way again.

Ricardo could no longer stand the suspense. He rejoined Flusher at Dacron's side and asked, "What is it, Doctor?"

Tears welled in her eyes. Unable to speak, she handed Ricardo the invoice that the technicians had left. It read, "Hard drive crashed. Irreparable damage. Consultation fee: $4233.50, payable 30 days net."

" 'Irreparable'?" Ricardo asked, not wanting to believe it. "Were they sure?"

Flusher nodded, blinking; tears spilled down her cheeks. She pulled out her handkerchief, blew her nose with it, then discarded it into a jar labeled STERILE GAUZE.

"But he's come back from the dead so many times," Ricardo persisted. Right off the top of his head Ricardo could recall several of them: the mission when Dacron went "down" and then revived once his program had cleared itself; the day Westerly saved Dacron by installing a new battery in his chest; and the many times Dacron's head had been blown off, misplaced, or removed as a practical joke, and eventually reattached. Ricardo added, "Surely someone who's been through all the things that Dacron has experienced should be able to come back from this."

Flusher shook her head. "Nobody survives a hard-drive crash." She began disconnecting the monitor electrodes from Dacron's chest. "If he'd been more careful about backing up his files on floppy disks every day, maybe we could reconstruct his programs," Flusher continued in a tone tempered with regret, "but that was the one area in which he always slacked off."

Tenderly she touched Dacron's shoulder. "He was so good about everything else . . . " she murmured, "eating a low-cholesterol diet . . . flossing . . . oil changes every three months . . . " Her voice drifted off.

Gazing at Dacron's lifeless form, Ricardo felt a stab of pain at the loss. *This means I'll have the tedious chore of interviewing people to take his place at the Oops station,* Ricardo thought. *What a bloody nuisance.*

Dacron had died while Ricardo and Flusher casually chatted at the sink in Sick Bay. His soul drifted out of his body and hovered in the operating area for a moment. Seeing that the Scramscope was about to set off an alarm that would have interrupted the conversation between Ricardo and Flusher, Dacron's soul thoughtfully disconnected the alarm mechanism.

Dacron realized that he was dead, and from his familiarity with the literature on near-death experience, he thought he knew exactly what to expect next. First, his soul would drift around the ship for a while. Then he would pass through a dark tunnel. Next he would see others who had died before him. Finally, he would confront a Being of Light, who would show him highlights of his lifetime and ask if he was ready to cross over into the afterlife.

However, Dacron soon discovered that near-death was a little different for an android. For one thing, his soul didn't hover near the ceiling the way most souls did. Instead, it scuttled along a few feet above the floor like a helium balloon that was past its prime. Every time somebody moved nearby, a draft of air sent Dacron's soul bobbing willy-nilly in another direction.

With his perspective limited to floor level, this phase of Dacron's experience was restricted to spotting dustballs and forgotten medical instruments dropped behind cabinets, although he did get one enlightening glimpse up Dr. Flusher's skirt. He was glad when the dark tunnel appeared, signaling the end of the tedious floating segment.

Dacron felt himself being sucked down the dark tunnel. It appeared much like a car tunnel on the freeway, and Dacron felt an overwhelming urge to honk his horn, then realized he didn't have one. Eventually he emerged on the other side of the tunnel.

Just as Dacron expected, there in the Great Beyond were others who had died before him, including Lull, the android daughter he'd constructed in his basement workshop, and Wart's old girlfriend K-Mart. Dacron tried to speak to them, but apparently they couldn't see or hear him. Something stood between him and the others, and Dacron surmised that he hadn't yet fully passed over into the afterlife.

Dacron looked around expectantly for the Being of Light,

that all-knowing, all-accepting power who would decide his final fate. But since Dacron was on the android track, he was met instead by the Being of Fluorescence.

Confronting the Being of Fluorescence wasn't exactly awe-inspiring. It was more like standing in the presence of a George Webb's all-night diner.

"Excuse me," Dacron said to the Being. "I am Dacron. I believe you are to show me the highlights of my life to help decide if my mission among the living has been accomplished."

The Being yawned, nodded, and flicked a hidden switch. Directly in front of them, clouds gathered to serve as a sort of motion picture screen, and Dacron's life was projected onto the clouds in a flickering 16mm film image. There were many boring scenes that consisted mainly of talking heads, with Dacron's head doing most of the talking, and the Being of Fluorescence fell asleep halfway through the story.

When it ended, the Being awoke with a start. Dacron, anticipating the Being's next action, said, "I believe you will now ask me whether I am prepared for the afterlife. Is that correct?"

"No," said the Being, getting up stiffly and turning off the lamp of the film projector. "I'm trying to decide whether or not to let you in. There's a quota on androids, so we decide on a case-by-case basis. Meanwhile, I'm going to have to put you on hold."

Before Dacron could protest, the Being flicked his hand, and instantly Dacron found himself in a doorless, windowless room. Another person sat on a bench in the corner, and Dacron recognized her at once: it was his deceased former crewmate Yasha Tar.

"Dacron! Fancy meeting you here," Yasha said. She was dressed in the Romanumen uniform in which she had appeared during her previous incarnation among the living.

"Yasha." Dacron studied their surroundings. "Where are we?"

She grinned, swept her arms wide, and said sarcastically,

"Welcome to Limbo. You sit here until it gets so dull back in the real world that they need you to juice things up. So you go back for a while, do a little song and dance, and when it's all over, you're yanked over here again."

Dacron seemed less than thrilled by the prospect. "This is not the career direction I envisioned for myself," he said.

Yasha wrinkled her mouth. "Me neither," she said. "But let's face it, Dacron. After six years of sitting at the Oops station, what else are you qualified to do?"

Dacron brightened. "I can sing," he replied. "My singing voice recently rose into the lyric soprano range. Would you like to hear a number?"

"Maybe later," Yasha told him. She patted the seat next to her. "C'mon and sit down. I want to hear all the news about what's happening on the other side."

That very night, Capt. Ricardo ordered that a funeral service for Dacron be held in an appropriate HolidayDeck setting. Ricardo believed that the others should face the reality of Dacron's death straight on, without delay. Besides, he didn't want the whole affair to drag out any longer, since it might mess up their Away Team mission the next morning.

Chief Engineer Georgie LaForgery painstakingly programmed the HolidayDeck to re-create a funeral-home parlor. Dacron's body was laid out in state at the front, and it was a sobering sight. His pale face matched the snowy white pillow on which his head rested. His hands, folded across his chest, clutched a sprig of air fern.

Bouquets of flowers surrounded the coffin, with banners bearing tribute to the many roles Dacron had filled: "Friend," "Crewmate" and "Major Shipboard Appliance." Even his estranged brother Lycra had sent a bouquet—apparently filched from a gravesite, judging from its faded plastic flowers and the legend VETERAN OF THE BORED WAR.

One by one, Dacron's crewmates stepped up to the coffin to pay their last respects.

Capt. Ricardo went first. Gazing at Dacron, he shook his

head with regret. "Dacron, Dacron," he murmured. "You're still so young. Why did you have to go so soon? Couldn't you have waited until the end of this mission?" Still shaking his head, Ricardo left the coffin and sat in one of the folding chairs to await the beginning of the memorial service.

Cmdr. Piker was next. He was beginning to show his age again as the fountain water wore off, and his somber expression made him look even more mature. "So long, old pal," Piker said softly to Dacron. "I'm going to miss staring at the back of your head on the Bridge all day."

Wart followed. He rested his hands on the edge of the coffin, gazed respectfully at Dacron for a long moment, then lifted his head straight up at the ceiling and let out a blood-curdling howl, scaring the wits out of the other mourners.

With a final respectful glance at Dacron, Wart stepped to the side. Piker said to him, "I thought that howling was a Kringle ritual to tell the dead that a Kringle warrior was about to join them. Why do it for Dacron?"

Wart grunted. "I wanted to warn those in the hereafter that a compulsive talker was coming into their midst," he replied. Then Wart turned to the Chief Mortician standing nearby and told him, "The body is now nothing but an empty shell. You may dispose of it as you wish."

"Er, thank you, sir," said the Chief Mortician. "I believe we'll stick with our original plan."

"Hmmmm. What plan is that?" Piker asked in idle curiosity. "Cremation? Or embalming, and then torpedoing him out into space?"

"No, sir," the mortician replied. He leaned closer to Piker and explained in a low tone, "With androids like Mr. Dacron, for whom the usual alternatives are inappropriate, we use . . . how can I put this delicately? . . . a TrashMasher."

Counselor Troit was next to step up to the coffin. Like Piker, she had begun aging again. Gone was the exhilaration of her brief respite from adulthood. Now her eyes brimmed with tears as she regarded the lifeless form of the android who had once captured her heart with his love letters and poetry, including some of the bawdiest limericks she'd ever read.

Troit leaned over to press a final kiss against Dacron's cheek. Unfortunately, she was unaware that his skin had cooled considerably; instantly her moist lips stuck to the superchilled hardness of his face.

The others stood at a distance awaiting their turn. Their indulgence toward Troit's sentimental gesture withered into distaste as the kiss seemed to go on and on. Guano muttered to Dr. Flusher, "Doesn't Emily Post say that it's improper to kiss the dead for longer than five seconds?" Flusher shrugged.

Troit waved her hands, trying to signal her predicament, but the others interpreted her fluttering fingers as an indication that the kiss was getting her all hot and bothered.

"Oh, gross!" Guano exclaimed. "Somebody ought to put a stop to this." The others, aghast, continued to do nothing but stare, so Guano took it on herself to end the spectacle. She marched toward the coffin and reached for Troit's arm. But before she could touch Troit, a splinter of light flashed next to her, and Q-Tip appeared.

"Well, well," Q-Tip said, taking in the entire funeral scene with a glance. "What have we here? A dead second officer. This looks like a job for the Quke continuum."

"Q-Tip," growled Capt. Ricardo, "this is no time for your foolishness. We are trying to have a solemn funeral here."

"Solemn, eh?" Q-Tip arched an eyebrow at Troit, whose lips were still plastered against Dacron's cheek. "Really, my dear, you should try to restrain yourself," Q-Tip chided her. "Where I come from, such practices are frowned upon." Troit tried to respond, but her biting retort came out as "Mmmm mmmm mmmmmm!"

Q-Tip turned back to Ricardo and continued, "Come, come, *mon Capuchin.* Perhaps now you'll strike a deal with me. You know I can bring your android back to life with a wave of my omnipotent hand. All I ask is that you grant the simple request I laid at your feet not long ago."

"I'm not going to bargain with you, Q-Tip," Ricardo retorted. "If I give in to you this once, there'll be no end to your demands."

"What was it that he asked, Captain?" Piker wanted to know. Ricardo glared at Q-Tip, refusing to answer.

"Captain, I know you like to stick to your principles and all that," Georgie broke in, "but Dacron's my best friend. Couldn't you bend the rules a little and give in to Q-Tip so we can have Dacron back?"

"What did he ask you to do?" Piker persisted. "Was it really something so terrible? Are we supposed to go annihilate an alien race or something? Bomb a space colony of orphans? What?"

"Captain," said Dr. Flusher, joining the fray, "if Dacron comes back to life, that's one less death on my medical record this year, and maybe my malpractice insurance won't go up after all."

Guano added, "Can't you please give in to him so we can have Dacron back?"

Troit, her lips still stuck on Dacron, moved her eyes meaningfully at Ricardo and urged, "Mmmmm mmmmm mmmmmm!"

"Captain, tell us," Piker insisted, "what does Q-Tip want you to do?"

Ricardo folded his arms across his chest and told them, "He wants me to give him a driving lesson on the *Endocrine*."

Immediately the air filled with their cries. "That's it?!" "Well, do it, then!" "I can't believe you'd let that stand in your way." "Just a driving lesson?"

"All right. All right," Ricardo said, holding up his hands for silence. "All right, Q-Tip," he conceded, "I'll give you your driving lesson if you'll bring Dacron back to life."

"Splendid!" Q-Tip exclaimed. He snapped his fingers, and immediately the two of them were transported to the Bridge— Q-Tip sitting at the Conn with Ricardo standing next to him.

"What about Dacron?" Ricardo asked.

"All in good time, *mon capon*," Q-Tip said. "I'll take care of him once the lesson is over. I want to make sure you follow through on this bargain. Now!" he went on, running his hands eagerly over the control console. "What comes first?"

"First you have to turn on the engine," said Ricardo, pointing to a button with a picture of a key on it. The engine turned over as soon as Q-Tip pressed the button.

"Now," Ricardo continued, "give it a little gas, keep your foot on the clutch, and move it out of 'park' into first gear—"

"Wait. Wait. You're telling me too much at once," Q-Tip complained. The ship lurched forward and died.

"You weren't giving it enough gas," Ricardo corrected him.

"But you said to give it just a little gas," Q-Tip protested. He restarted the engine and tried again.

Five false starts later, Q-Tip managed to get the ship moving forward.

"Steer a straight course," Ricardo told him. "Look in the mirror so you know what's around you. Glance over your shoulder at your blind spot, too."

"You're talking too fast again," Q-Tip whined, clutching the console nervously. He glanced back over his shoulder as instructed. "What blind spot?" he asked.

"Look out for that meteor!" Ricardo shouted. He shoved Q-Tip's arm aside and pressed the steering buttons; the ship swerved, missing the meteor by mere feet.

"Hey," Q-Tip protested, trying to pry Ricardo's hands off the console, "this is my turn to drive, not yours."

Reluctantly Ricardo let go of the controls. A few seconds later, the ship began to bounce violently.

"What's that?" Q-Tip demanded, his face turning white with fear.

"Turbulence," Ricardo said, grabbing the back of Q-Tip's chair to keep his balance. "Try to steer around it—whoa!"

The ship hit an air pocket and plunged several thousand feet. It finally bottomed out in a landing that felt like hitting solid rock. The turbulence resumed, bouncing them repeatedly.

"Wh-uh-uh-what duh-uh-uh-uh-do I-I-I du-uh-uh-do?" Q-Tip asked as his chin struck his chest again and again.

Back in the HolidayDeck funeral parlor, the others rode out the swaying and bouncing of the ship during Q-Tip's driving lesson. Wart, Piker and Georgie braced themselves against Dacron's casket so it wouldn't tip over. Guano managed to free Troit's lips from Dacron's cheek by heating the contact point with the blow-dryer she always carried around in her hat.

Finally the wild ride smoothed out. A few minutes later, Q-Tip and Ricardo re-entered the funeral parlor, caught up in a bitter argument.

"You call that driving instruction?" Q-Tip sputtered. "I'm not even ready to get my learner's permit after that travesty."

"You asked for a first lesson, and that's exactly what I gave you," Ricardo replied.

"I didn't ask for a first lesson," Q-Tip hissed. "I asked you to teach me to drive. I wanted to learn freeway merging, parallel parking, the whole enchilada."

"You got what we agreed on," Ricardo insisted. "Now hold up your side of the bargain. Bring Dacron back to life."

"What you gave me wasn't what we agreed on," Q-Tip retorted. "It was just your interpretation of what we agreed on—a flagrant piece of creative finagling. Well, two can play that game. You want Dacron brought back to life? Fine! But I'm going to do it *my* way!"

Still glaring at Ricardo, Q-Tip snapped his fingers at Dacron. Dacron blinked a couple of times and started to stir. The others, filled with joy and relief, gathered around his coffin.

"Dacron, can you hear me?" Dr. Flusher asked.

Slowly, a sultry smile spread across Dacron's face. "Hullo, darlin'," he drawled.

Hands reached out to help Dacron sit up. "You were pretty far gone there for a while," Flusher continued. "You went down when I tried to re-orient your circuits. Everything seems to be in order now."

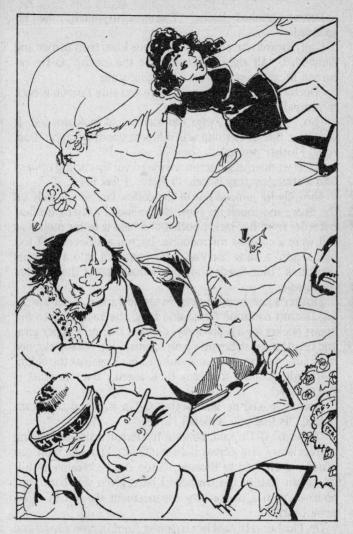

The others rode out the swaying and bouncing of the ship.

Dacron blinked lazily. "Thangyouvurymuch," he responded.

Capt. Ricardo gave Dacron a dubious look, then turned and demanded, "All right, Q-Tip, what's the catch?" Q-Tip returned Ricardo's stare with a taunting smile.

"Doctor," Ricardo continued, "are you sure Dacron is back to normal?"

"No," said Flusher, who was starting to look worried. It was clear that something was different about Dacron. "Dacron," Flusher prompted, "how do you feel?"

"I feel wunnerful," Dacron answered, his lip curling upward into a strangely sexy twitch. "I feel . . . I feel like . . . "

Abruptly he jumped out of the coffin, landed squarely on the floor, and shook his hips. He grabbed Flusher's medical tricorder from her jacket pocket and held it to his mouth as if it were a cordless microphone. Dacron announced, "I feel like singin' a song for y'all." He launched into a raucous version of "Blue Suede Shoes" in a husky tenor that befitted the classic.

Flusher's jaw dropped open in astonishment. After watching Dacron continue for several bars, she reached into her breast pocket for a hippospray, grabbed Dacron's upper arm, and thrust the instrument firmly against him. Dacron stopped his frantic performance and slumped back against the coffin.

Ricardo, helping to steady him, asked, "Dacron, what is the matter?"

Dacron looked up and, seeing Q-Tip standing there, inquired, "Is that you, Colonel Parker?"

"Indeed," Q-Tip said, coming to Dacron's side and laying a proprietary arm across his shoulders. "You see, *mon cap pistol*," Q-Tip said to Ricardo, "I too can be creative in fulfilling my half of the bargain. I have given you back your android, with a personality enhancement thrown in at no extra charge."

Dr. Flusher retrieved her tricorder from Dacron's hand and passed it over his head and chest to check his vital signs.

"Dacron," she said, "I'm so sorry to have put you through all this. I sincerely hope you won't sue me for malpractice."

"Ah forgive yuh, baby," Dacron said with a smile, cocking a languorous eyebrow at Flusher. "But puh-*lease* stop callin' me 'Dacron.' Muh name's Elvis, honey."

6

The Wrong Arm
of the Law

THE NEXT MORNING, before heading over to help open the park, Capt. Smirk visited Mr. Smock, who was monitoring the sensors on the Bridge of the *Endocrine*.

"What d'ya think, Smock? Is it catchy enough?" Smirk asked, holding up a t-shirt for Smock's inspection. Imprinted on the front of the shirt was the legend JUVEN ISLE: THE HAPPIEST PLACE IN THE GALAXY.

Smirk continued eagerly, "This shirt is just a prototype, but we can have fifteen thousand of 'em sewn up in about a week. The sales rep said that anything made out of this fabric sells like crazy. It turns different colors when you're horny. Look!" Smirk held the t-shirt against his chest, and the tie-dyed pattern began flashing in neon hues.

Smock gave it his impassive once-over. "Very eye-catching," he judged.

"I gotta go," Smirk said, turning on his heel and heading for the door. "There's a big group comin' in this morning, and I hafta make sure the ticket takers are ready." Smirk had already marketed a group rate for park admissions, and the Born to Be Wild Intergalactic Reform School for Girls was the first to take advantage of it.

"Captain," Smock called after him, "before you go, I believe you should be aware of a message the sensors picked up last night. We have a recording of it."

Smirk stepped back to Smock's station, and Smock told him, "This was an audio transmission from Admiral Less at

Starfreak Headquarters to a field commander named Bungeeman Crisco." Smock pressed the "replay" button on his console.

The recording began with Crisco's groggy voice. "Huh... hullo?" he said.

"Crisco? This is Admiral Less at Starfreak Headquarters." Even in a recording, her voice was as piercing as a dentist's drill. "You sound funny, Crisco. Do you have a cold or something?"

"Unhh... no..." Bedsprings creaked in the background. "It's just that I was asleep when you called, Admiral."

"Asleep? Hmmm. Well, it's time you got up anyway. I want you to start on a new mission immediately." Briefly, Admiral Less filled him in on Starfreak's intention to oust Smirk, claim the Fountain of Youth, and transport Smirk's crew to the nursing home.

"We'd sent somebody else on this mission, but he blew it," she concluded crisply. "I don't want to waste any more time on this. Get in there and get the job done."

"Yes, Admiral," Crisco responded.

Mr. Smock broke in. "The remainder of their conversation is merely routine," he said, turning off the recording. He went on, "I calculated the probable coordinates of Commander Crisco's ship when he received this message. Allowing for travel at the average cruising speed of Warped 8.23, he should arrive here today at approximately 0900 hours. Do you wish to take any countermeasures against him, Captain?"

"No, Smock," Smirk replied. "His crew will probably come looking for us in the park. Don't try to keep them from Faxing down here. We'll just let them, like, roam around. Once they hit the water of Juven Isle, they'll lighten up—big time."

Aboard Capt. Ricardo's orbiting ship that morning, Counselor Troit was having a difficult time getting out of bed. And no wonder: the previous day at suppertime, she'd been a sprightly 15-year-old, and now she was attempting to arise and shine after gaining 20 years overnight. The Fountain of Youth water had definitely worn off.

This was not just a normal case of the early-morning blahs. This mother of all rude awakenings was like a humongous boulder of Elmer's Glue-All that pressed her against the mattress and oozed around her ears.

With enormous effort, Troit opened her eyes. Dimly she wondered how in the world that 15-year-old body had managed to cram so much living into the past few days. Now she was paying for it; every single muscle either ached or had gone on strike.

She forced herself out of bed to get ready for an early-morning counseling session; Capt. Ricardo had asked her to debrief Dacron regarding his near-death experience.

Meanwhile, in his own quarters, Cmdr. Piker was suffering a similar case of the Monday-morning syndrome. His beard had yet to grow back, but everything else about him had deteriorated from factory-fresh condition to somewhat-worse-for-the-wear during the night.

Capt. Ricardo, on the other hand, had sprung out of bed extra early to allow time for a project he'd been putting off: investigating what Wart was up to. In fact, all the mental notes Ricardo had been making about this project were accumulating into a full-length symphony. And another incident had arisen to suggest that Ricardo should check out the situation soon.

When the Away Team had returned to the ship the previous night, there'd been a memo on Ricardo's desk from the principal of the *Endocrine*'s day school. She'd complained that Wart's private school had beaten the day-school team in a game of tackle football, even though Wart's school had only one pupil in it. Apparently Smartalecsander had shown no mercy on the other kids.

As he approached Wart's quarters, Ricardo noticed that the handmade sign at the door had been replaced by a permanent plaque that read KRINGLE MILITARY ACADEMY / ABANDON ALL HOPE, YE WHO ENTER HERE.

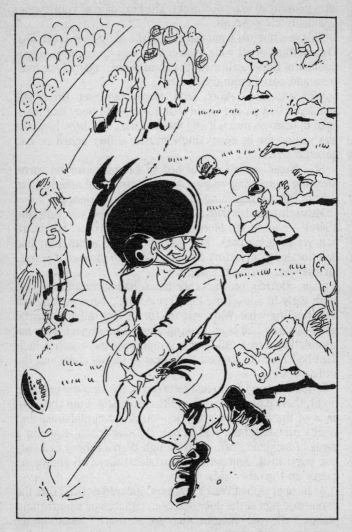

Smartalecsander had shown no mercy on the other kids.

Ricardo rang the door chime. "Come in," he heard Wart say.

Wart and Smartalecsander were seated at the dining table. "Captain," said Wart, standing to greet him and indicating a vacant chair. "Please, sit down."

"Mr. Wart," Ricardo began as he took the seat, "shouldn't Smartalecsander be attending classes with the rest of the children?"

Wart stiffened. "I am teaching my son myself, Captain," he replied. "In fact, we are having a lesson right now." Ricardo glanced at Smartalecsander, who was simply eating from a dinner plate.

Noticing Ricardo's skepticism, Wart explained, "It is a lesson in discipline. Smartalecsander is to finish that serving of brussels sprouts without whining or gagging."

"I see," said Ricardo. "Wart, I understand your desire to raise Smartalecsander in the Kringle tradition. But the Starfreak Board of Education has certain standards. Homeschooled children aren't considered properly educated. For that reason, when they get older, they are seldom admitted to Starfreak Academy."

Wart looked perturbed; the wrinkles on his forehead knotted into a tangle. "I was not aware of that," he admitted.

"I'm sure you want that option to remain open for your son," Ricardo added. "Admission to Starfreak Academy is the highest goal a student can aspire to."

Smartalecsander, sensing that the balance of power was shifting, stopped eating his brussels sprouts. Immediately Wart prompted him, "Eat your vegetables, young man." Craftily, Smartalecsander continued forking the green globules into his mouth, ever so slowly, but he stopped chewing them.

Capt. Ricardo said, "I'll never forget my own days at the Academy. I gained a lifetime's worth of knowledge there. In fact, some of the best lessons came outside of the classroom."

Wart shifted impatiently in his chair. Like all the senior officers, he'd heard the story of Ricardo's school days a million times. Sitting beside Wart, Smartalecsander slowed his fork motion even further while squirreling away another brussels sprout in his cheek.

"One mentor in particular stands out," Ricardo went on. "He was an old gardener named Toothby."

Wart barely suppressed a groan. Smartalecsander shoved another brussels sprout into his mouth and faked a chewing motion.

"Toothby was a retired Martian who'd taken the gardening job to supplement his Social Security income. Though he wasn't a scholar, he possessed an abundance of another kind of knowledge," Ricardo said, leaning back in his chair and warming to the story. "I used to follow him as he worked, and occasionally, if I were lucky, he would let me scatter manure around the flower beds. By the time I was a sophomore, he even let me borrow his shovel for the job. In the spring of my senior year, I helped him spread Milorganite over the lawn. Ah, those were glorious days."

A low rumble of impatience emerged from Wart's chest; he couldn't help himself. Smartalecsander, studying his father's face, realized that Wart was near the breaking point. The boy stopped all pretense of chewing.

Ricardo recalled, "Toothby used to say to me, 'Jean-Lucy, gardening is like life. If things aren't going your way, just dump another load of manure over everything around you.' It's a lesson I use in my command every day. In fact—"

"AAARRRGGGGHHHH!" Wart erupted. He jumped up as if to engage in battle, then caught himself and stood there panting heavily. "All right, you win!" he shouted. "Just stop talking about Toothby!"

Ricardo, taken aback for a moment, quickly recovered and asked Wart, "You mean you're willing to send Smartalecsander back to day school?"

"Yes," Wart conceded.

Smartalecsander, realizing that this last lesson in discipline at the Kringle Military Academy could go unfinished, promptly opened his jaw to its widest and disgorged a pile of brussels sprouts onto his plate.

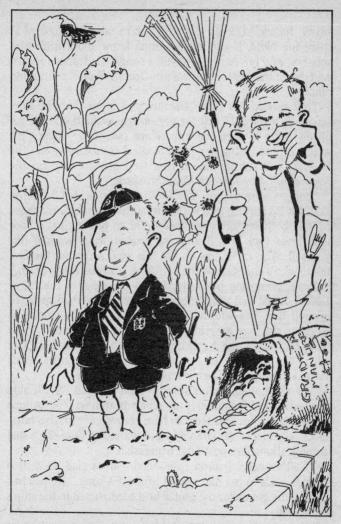

"If I were lucky, he would let me scatter manure around the flower beds."

* * *

"Aww, honey," Dacron drawled, "ah'm tahr'd of lookin' at these ink blots. If yuh really wanna know about muh personality, why not let me sing yuh a song?" He leaned forward eagerly on the edge of the sofa in Deanna Troit's counseling office.

Troit pursed her lips. "Dacron, you know that the Rorschach is a standard test for personality evaluation," she replied, trying to keep the impatience out of her voice. "It's well accepted within the psychological community, and the findings will substantiate my writeup of your case for the *Journal of Serendipitous Headshrinkery*."

"Baby, you're makin' this way too complicated," Dacron said, his lip curling into a half-smile that somehow managed to look both sensuous and sweet. "Ah'm just a good ol' boy who loves rock-'n'-roll and appreciates pretty women like yourself. Who cares how ah got this way? Ah'm not the first felluh who's changed for the bettuh after a brush with death."

Troit, glimpsing her reflection in the glass of the coffee table, noticed that a faint network of crow's feet had sprouted around her eyes within the last half hour. She wondered whether she was suffering a rebound as the fountain water wore off; maybe she'd end up older than she'd been to start with. The thought left her too dispirited to continue this formal inquiry into Dacron's personality quirks.

"All right, then, never mind," Troit allowed. "We'll skip the tests, and I'll construct my report from field observations of your behavior. You seem to have recovered from this near-death experience remarkably well, without any of the usual complications like post-fatal depression."

"That's swell," Dacron responded. "Ah'm glad we settled that. Sounds to me like a good time for a song." He reached behind the couch for the guitar he'd constructed in the ship's replicator.

"Not now, Dacron," Troit told him. "Dr. Flusher asked me to send you to Sick Bay after we'd finished our session. She wants you to undergo a medical evaluation before our away mission."

Dacron nodded and prepared to leave. "She's gonna love the new me," he predicted. "Ah've noticed that muh entire body is so much more flexible. Especially muh hips."

Capt. Ricardo and Wart dropped off Smartalecsander at the *Endocrine*'s schoolroom and headed for Shipping and Receiving, where the Away Team would meet to Fax down to the amusement park once again. Halfway down the hall, they were joined by Guano the bartender.

She'd dressed casually for a day of fun and games. Instead of her usual voluminous robe, she wore a baseball jersey over bike shorts.

As the three of them stepped into the Crewmover, Ricardo gave her the once-over and remarked, "Guano, this is an official mission. We're not visiting the park to enjoy ourselves. There are no side trips allowed."

"You mean I won't even be able to buy souvenirs?" Guano whined. Capt. Ricardo shook his head. "Then I guess I won't be needing this extra money," Guano concluded, tipping her head toward the floor. Out of the top of her enormous hat, a sheaf of currency floated to the floor, and coins clanked and rattled and bounced out. Guano held out her jersey like an apron and scooped up all the money into it.

The Crewmover doors opened, and Guano walked out first, heading for the public lockers at the side of the Shipping bay. She put a quarter into one of them, pulled out the key, dumped her money inside, and shut it for safekeeping.

Troit and Piker were already in Shipping, standing near the UltraFax platform. Piker, holding out his arms pleadingly, was asking Troit, "Look, all I want to know is, are we still going steady?" Troit shrugged.

Ricardo walked over to Dr. Flusher, who was waiting next to the UltraFax control panel with Chief Engineer Georgie LaForgery. "Is Q-Tip still around?" Ricardo asked Flusher.

"The last time I saw him, he was looking through the window of Sick Bay, watching you examine Dacron."

Flusher shook her head and said, "Q-Tip is gone. He spent some time revamping Dacron's wardrobe, and then he left the ship."

"Where is Dacron?" Ricardo continued. "Have you and Counselor Troit decided whether he's well enough to come with us on this mission?"

Flusher nodded. "Yes, he is. He's waiting just around the corner in the hall," she told the captain. "He said he wanted to make a big entrance once the whole Away Team gets here."

"Well, the rest of us are ready to go," said Ricardo, glancing around impatiently.

As if on cue, the door from the hallway swooshed open, and Dacron jumped into the room. He was a different Dacron than they were used to. Among androids, now he was clearly The King.

Gone was his minimalist swept-back hairdo; in its place was a dramatic mane that cascaded over his forehead. Thick wooly sideburns accented his cheeks. His yellow eyes were camouflaged by sunglasses that gave him an air of utter cool.

A cluster of gold chains glittered at his neck. The top three buttons of his shirt collar were unbuttoned, revealing a shock of chest hair that hadn't been there yesterday, and the back of his collar was turned up rakishly.

Dacron spread his arms wide in a gesture of showmanship. The rhinestones on his hiphuggers caught the light.

The crew stared at him. Finally Georgie recovered a little from the initial shock and politely applauded Dacron's entrance.

Rings glistened on every finger as Dacron held a Mr. Microphone to his lips. "Thangyouvurymuch," he said, acknowledging Georgie's applause. "Ah wanna do a little number for yuh now that ah think you're gonna like."

Dacron pressed a button on the microphone. It must have been a remote control, for out of nowhere, background music immediately began blaring a rowdy but somehow familiar tune. Dacron sang:

> You ain't nothin' but a Pakled
> Droolin' all the time.
> You ain't nothin' but a Pakled
> Droolin' all the time.
> You may own a lotta hardware
> But your brain ain't worth a dime.

Then the music changed; the first few bars of "I Can't Help Falling in Love with You" wafted forth. "Ah'm gonna slow it down a little now," Dacron told his audience.

But before Dacron could shift into the ballad, Ricardo stopped him. "That's enough, Dacron," Ricardo ordered, grabbing the microphone and turning off the background music.

Ricardo led them onto the UltraFax platform. Dacron, somewhat subdued, followed in his usual obedient manner, though he did swivel his hips while waiting on the pad.

Not far from Ricardo's *Endocrine*, another craft approached the planet and prepared to assume orbiting altitude. At its helm was Cmdr. Bungeeman Crisco.

Crisco's physical appearance revealed that he was well on the way to following the trend set by Capt. Ricardo—prepared to *baldly* go where nobody wanted to go before.

This mission to transport Smirk & Co. to the Vacant Attic struck Crisco as so laughably easy that he hadn't even bothered to bring along any of his Starfreak subordinates. He'd simply borrowed a paddywagon craft and carried a phaser set on "gentle stun." From what Admiral Less had told him, Crisco didn't expect Smirk and his officers to put up much resistance.

"You'll know them when you see them," Admiral Less had assured Crisco after giving him his orders. "Relics. Ready for the fox farm."

Although Crisco hadn't been too keen on being awakened in the middle of the night by Admiral Less' call, once he got going on the mission, he felt a stirring of hope. Maybe this was the fresh start he needed, for he'd been having a run of bad luck lately.

First his wife Hennypenny was killed aboard the *Sara Lee* when the evil machine-like Bored started recycling all the metal in the starship without bothering to remove the crew and passengers first. Crisco's last-minute escape from the imploding ship with his son Joke still gave him nightmares, especially when he thought about the autographed Babe Ruth jockstrap he'd been forced to leave behind.

Starfreak's life insurance carrier refused to honor Crisco's claim on Hennypenny's policy; they maintained that a death ray emanating from a giant metal cube was considered an act of God. Then came the most crushing blow: Crisco's hairline began receding about a half-inch per day for no apparent reason. "Stress," the doctors diagnosed, telling him to take two hipposprays and call them at the turn of the century.

The ironic twist was that part of the blame for his wife's death could be traced to a fellow Starfreak officer—a traitor who had aided and abetted the Bored in their attempt to take over the universe. Crisco, like everyone else in the federation, knew that some captain named Jean-Lucy Ricardo had been captured and was temporarily turned into a half-machine Bored.

The Bored, master recyclers that they were, had picked Ricardo's brain for every useful bit of Starfreak military strategy they could find amidst the reams of Shakespearean dialogue, archeological writings and alien-flute solos. The Bored used this military strategy against the federation in the Bored War. With Ricardo—renamed "Lowcutie"—leading them, they'd destroyed scores of federation ships and killed thousands of people. True, they'd done it against Ricardo's will, and afterward he'd said he was really, awfully sorry, but the damage was already done.

A glance at the control screen of Crisco's shuttlecraft

brought his wandering thoughts back to his current mission. Sensors indicated that there was already a starship orbiting the planet where he was headed—undoubtedly Smirk's ship, Crisco figured. He steered clear of it, pulled into an empty orbit path, shifted his shuttle into "park," and turned off the engine. After a final check of the sensors, which clearly outlined the inhabited areas of the surface, Crisco set the shuttle's UltraFax on auto mode and Faxed himself down.

"What is it, Smock?" responded Smirk, addressing the intercom in the ceiling of his management office. Smock had just hailed him from the Bridge of their ship in the parking lot. "Make it short. I'm busy," Smirk added, with a suave smile at the young woman sitting on his lap.

"Captain, Commander Crisco just entered orbit and Faxed down to the entrance gate," came Smock's voice. "I thought you would like to be informed."

"Thank you, Smock," Smirk responded. He smoothed back a curl on his companion's forehead. "I'll track him with the surveillance camera monitors."

Smirk's eyes never quite made it to the monitors. If they had, though, he would have seen Crisco pass by Smirk's officers one by one, totally unaware that these youngsters in their jaunty park uniforms were his intended prey.

Three hours later, Cmdr. Crisco, tired and cranky from fighting the crowds of Juven Isle, decided to take a break and assess his options.

He hadn't spotted anyone who looked remotely like an aging Starfreak officer. The vast majority of those crowding the park were exuberant young patrons who charged at top speed from one ride to the next, jostling Crisco and stepping on his toes en route.

It was near noon, and Crisco realized he hadn't eaten in quite a while. He headed for the nearest fast-food restaurant, a pizza joint decorated to look like an old-fashioned firehouse. There was a long wait in the line to order food, so he had plenty of time to study the carefully arranged details of the firehouse decor, including moldy firehoses hanging on the walls, worn rubber boots standing as centerpieces on each table, and a Dalmatian that wandered around begging for table scraps.

Finally Crisco got his cola and a slice of greasy pizza. He scanned the room for a table, but every place was filled.

Wandering through the dining area with his paper plate and cup, Crisco spotted a doorway which looked like it might lead to another seating area. As he drew near, though, he realized that this was a small banquet room that seemed to be fully occupied. A few steps closer and he noticed that the diners were wearing Starfreak uniforms. Immediately he slid to one side of the doorway to avoid drawing attention to himself.

Crisco approached the entrance sidewise. A lone dining chair was placed just outside the door; he sat on it, cocking his ear toward the opening.

"Mr. Chairman," said someone inside, "I want to call the question."

"You can't call the question," said another voice. "There's already a motion on the floor to amend the previous motion."

"Well, then," said the first voice, "I move we get that motion off the floor and take a vote to call the answer."

Crisco felt a nudge at his knee. The Dalmatian was sniffing at the plate of pizza in his lap. Crisco lifted the plate and shook his foot at the dog, whispering, "Shoo! Shoo!"

The dog persisted, whining a little and scratching at Crisco's pants leg. "Quiet, boy," Crisco hissed, swinging an elbow at the dog while balancing his pizza in one hand and his cola in the other.

The discussion in the next room was getting louder. "You know," someone observed, "we started this meeting an hour ago and we still haven't gotten past the motion to accept the minutes of the last meeting."

"All in good time, Number 1," said another. "There is no substitute for proper procedure."

Crisco wondered, *Who are these guys? Could this be Smirk and his crew? They certainly sound like retirees—like they've got all the time in the world.* Crisco's heart raced as he speculated, *Maybe this detour to the pizza parlor has led me straight to my targets.*

The dog at his elbow whined louder. "Shhh!" Crisco responded. He tried holding the plate higher, but still the dog managed to lick the crust. In desperation, Crisco raised the plate and carefully placed it atop his own head. This broad, smooth platform held the pizza out of the Dalmatian's reach. With his newly freed hand, Crisco pulled out his phaser. Carefully he stood up and leaned close to the doorway.

Someone was saying, "I move we amend the motion to table the question that called the answer."

Another voice added, "And I want to attach a rider that says we'll approach the management office with phasers on 'maximum stun.' "

"You can't attach a rider unless the person who made the motion agrees," countered someone else, "and you have to call out 'Simon says' before you do it."

Warily, Crisco peered around the corner. He spotted a bald Starfreak officer at the head of the table; the insignia on his collar indicated that he was a captain. *This has to be Smirk and his crew,* Crisco decided. *No wonder Starfreak wants to put them out to pasture. What a bunch of fuddy-duddys.*

Unexpectedly, the Dalmatian, frustrated that Crisco's food remained out of reach, whined piercingly and gave a series of short yelps. The captain turned toward the door, asking, "What was that?" In the nick of time, Crisco pulled back from the doorframe.

This is it, Crisco thought. *Time to make my move.*

He thrust the phaser forward and leaped into the room. "Freeze!" he ordered. "You're all under arrest!" Eight Starfreak crewmembers stared back at him. At first their expressions showed pure surprise, but then a few smiled and even giggled; and Crisco realized he was still balancing the plate of pizza on his head and holding the cola in his other hand.

Holding the phaser at readiness, he set the cola on the table, then carefully retrieved the pizza from its platform and set it down too.

The Dalmatian seized the chance—lunged forward, snatched the slice of pizza, and darted out of the room.

The bald captain at the head of the table asked in an icy tone, "Would you mind telling us what this is all about, *Commander*?" He gave the title a slight but unmistakable twist of derision.

"I'm Commander Bungeeman Crisco," came the reply, "and by order of Admiral Less of Starfreak Command, I'm taking you under arrest and transporting you to the Vacant Attic Nursing Home." Crisco was so hyper from the thrill of making this arrest that he failed to notice that most of the crewmembers were well under retirement age.

"The Vacant Attic? Us?" The captain looked confused for a moment; then his expression cleared. "Ah," he said, "you must have mistaken us for Captain Smirk's crew."

"Don't try to pull any fast ones on me," Crisco growled. "I know that's just who you are." He cranked the phaser up from "gentle stun" to the "major owie" setting, making sure everyone saw him do it.

Even at such close proximity, Crisco still failed to recognize Ricardo as Lowcutie, the Bored who'd appeared on the Viewscreen of the *Sara Lee* ordering them to surrender. During that encounter, half of Ricardo's face had been obscured by a metal plate in the Bored's "Foundry Chic" fashion style.

"All right, hands on the table," Crisco ordered. Reluctantly, they all complied, and Crisco circled them, confiscating their phasers. Then he went around the table again and began frisking each of them for additional weapons.

"But I'm not Captain Smirk," the captain protested. "Actually, I'm here to capture him, just as you are. I'm Captain Jean-Lucy Ricardo."

"Yeah, and I'm Pope Priscilla XIII," Crisco snarled. He spent a few extra moments frisking Counselor Troit's curves. *You can't be too careful with these renegades*, he told himself.

Crisco moved on to frisk Dacron. Running his hands roughly over the android's back, he unknowingly flicked the "off" switch, and Dacron collapsed onto the table. Appalled at Dacron's sudden apparent demise, Crisco jumped back and gasped, "Ohmygosh."

Troit, rolling her eyes in exasperation, leaned over and reset the switch. Dacron re-booted, looking a little groggy, with his sideburns slightly askew. "Whoa, mama," he slurred. "Did somebody get the number of th' truck that hit me?"

"No, really," the captain persisted. "I am Captain Jean-Lucy Ricardo."

Crisco whirled around to face the captain and pointed the phaser directly at his head. "Look, cut out this baloney sausage," he warned. "I know you're James T. Smirk. Don't keep bringing up the name of this Ricardo guy, 'cause that traitor was responsible for the death of my wife during the Bored War."

The bald captain gulped, apparently alarmed at Crisco's fierceness.

"So if you *were* Ricardo," Crisco continued, "I'd pull your tonsils up from your throat and wrap them in a bow around your skull. As it is, I'm just going to take you into custody and dump you at the nursing home."

Crisco backed away a few steps and ordered, "All right, everybody up." He herded them into a group and began setting his remote Fax control. "You'll sit in a detention cell on my shuttlecraft during the trip," he told them. "I'll be pulling your ship with a tractor beam. This will be a no-frills ride, so don't expect any complimentary soft drinks or peanuts on the way there."

As they stood waiting to be Faxed up, Piker, who was just outside of Crisco's earshot, murmured, "Captain Ricardo, aren't we going to fight back?"

"What can we do?" the captain whispered in response. "Besides, I think fighting back in this instance would violate the Prime Time Directive. And stop bringing up the name

'Ricardo,' " he added, nervously fingering his throat. "From now on, call me Captain Smirk."

The clerk at the reception desk of the Vacant Attic Nursing Home looked up expectantly as Crisco escorted Ricardo's crew through the front door. "Oooh!" she squealed. "You must be Captain Smirk and his group. We've been waiting for you." She reached for her phone receiver, pressed a button on the phone's base, and spoke over the public-address system: "Escorts to the front desk, please."

Crisco stepped up to the counter. The receptionist told him, "We'll just need to fill out some papers to make everything official." With considerable effort, she hefted a two-foot-high stack of papers onto the counter. Consulting the first form, she began, "Are the residents bringing any vehicles for the storage yard?"

"Just one," Crisco replied, "a Galahad-class starship, registry number NBC 1701 D-minus." The clerk wrote the number on a plastic tag and handed it to Crisco.

"Hang this from the front mirror," she instructed, "and pull the vehicle around the back to Lot A. That's where our residents keep their cars, RVs, Harley-Davidson cycles and so on. When they're not using them, of course."

Crisco figured that most of the vehicles probably stayed in mint condition. None of the residents in this lobby, at least, were about to take them out for a spin; they sat dozing in the upholstered chairs, warmed by the midafternoon sun streaming through the windows.

The escorts who had been summoned by the p.a. appeared in the lobby. Each of them took charge of one crewmember.

"Hello," said one of them, greeting Ricardo loudly and with exaggerated enunciation. "How are we feeling today?"

" 'We' are fine, and not the least bit deaf," he replied tartly.

"Oh, my," she responded with a tolerant chuckle. "Somebody hasn't had his prunes for breakfast, has he? We'll have to get you in a jolly mood. You can sit in on my canasta club this afternoon."

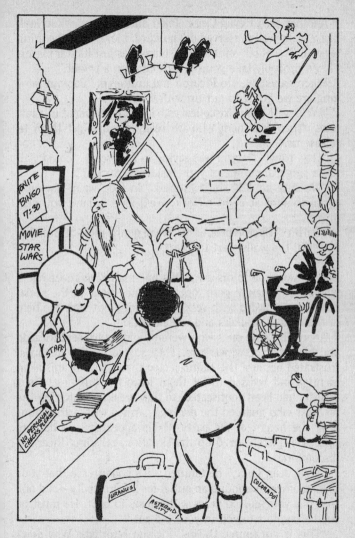

Crisco stepped up to the counter.

Another escort eyed Cmdr. Piker and observed, "You look like a really well-preserved old buzzard. I know just the thing for you. One of our shuffleboard teams has lost its star player. They'd probably take you on without even a tryout."

Piker leaned over to Ricardo and muttered, "Captain, how long are we going to put up with this?"

"We'll wait until Crisco leaves," Ricardo answered in a low tone, "then tell them who we really are and get them to release us."

"Hey, baby," Dacron was saying to his escort, "could y'all use a singer for some of your residents' parties?"

"We sure could!" she twittered. "In fact, we're having a social tonight at eight o'clock. We'd love to have you perform."

"Darlin'," Dacron promised, "we're gonna rock- 'n'-roll this place till the walls start to sweat."

Dacron was true to his word. His one-man Elvis revue had a whole lotta shakin' goin' on. The dance floor of the social room was crowded with residents rocking out with the help of their canes, walkers and wheelchairs.

About the only ones who weren't joining in were Ricardo and his other crewmembers. They sulked on the sidelines, frustrated because the staff rejected their claim of mistaken identity and refused to let them leave the building. Their phasers had been confiscated, so they were no match for the bouncer who guarded the doorway, armed with a stun gun.

At the height of the party, Q-Tip appeared in a flash of light. He quickly sized up the situation, relishing Ricardo's discomfort.

"Well, Jean-Lucy," he taunted, "it's good to see that your second officer has found an outlet for his creativity—and one that fills your golden years with music to boot. He must be such a comfort to you in your old age."

"This is not funny, Q-Tip," Ricardo retorted. "Why don't you put your powers to good use and get us out of here?"

Q-Tip didn't seem to hear him. He was studying Dacron and the wild party scene with increasing interest.

"You know, that boy really knows how to rock," he mused, almost to himself. "They're crazy about him." Onstage, Dacron removed the scarf from his neck and wiped his sweaty face with it, drawing squeals of delight from the female residents.

The number ended, and Dacron announced a short intermission. He started to stroll toward his crewmates but moved just a few feet beyond the stage before being mobbed by fans.

Q-Tip nodded and said to no one in particular, "Yes. Let's do it." He snapped his fingers, and both he and Dacron vanished in beams of dazzling light. The fans looked around in bewilderment when Dacron disappeared, but since none of them had much short-term memory to speak of, their disappointment was brief. Within moments they were stampeding toward the refreshment table, having completely forgotten about The King's *concert interruptus*.

A few minutes later there was another flash of light, and Q-Tip and Dacron reappeared at Ricardo's side. "Jean-Lucy, my protégé has something he'd like to tell you," said Q-Tip, flashing a triumphant grin.

Dacron shook back the shock of hair that had fallen across his eyes and asked his crewmates, "Have y'all met muh manager, Colonel Parker?" He indicated Q-Tip with a wave of his hand. "The colonel has some great plans for muh career. He's gonna take me out on tour, get me a recordin' contract, and even have me do some movies. So ah guess ah'll be out on the road for awhile. It's been nice workin' with y'all. Ah'll be sure to come back for a visit someday."

"Dacron, have you lost your mind?" Capt. Ricardo protested, but there was yet another flash of light, and Dacron and Q-Tip disappeared.

7

Hello Muddah,
Hello Faddah

Mercenary Caregivers Ltd.
"Your deterioration is our business"
Administrators of quality nursing homes:
Vacant Attic • Love 'Em & Leave 'Em
Stow 'N' Go • Forgotten but Not Gone
Nevermore • Last Gasp

MEMO

To: Vacant Attic Nursing Home Resident
#5482992, Capt. James T. Smirk, a.k.a. "Capt.
Jean-Lucy Ricardo"

From: Gareth Flintbottom, MD, Ph.D, Maitre D'—
Administrator, Mercenary Caregivers Ltd.

RE: Your letter of Stardate 38285.2¼

Your recent letter to our administrative headquarters, regarding the so-called "confusion" of your identity, has been forwarded to my office.

If it pleases you to be called "Jean-Lucy Ricardo"
rather than James T. Smirk (which was your officially registered name upon check-in), then our staff
will be happy to oblige, just as they did for your second officer, "Elvis." As you know, we always try to

humor any request of our residents, as long as it doesn't cost us anything.

However, I am afraid you are nowhere near ready for release from the Vacant Attic Nursing Home. You must rid yourself of this notion. I suggest you stay busy to help you keep your mind off the matter. Perhaps you could join your facility's craft guild and begin an apprenticeship in basketweaving.

Starfreak Command
Headquarters Building
Office #2292N

Dear <u>Capt. Ricardo</u>   :
    Thank you for your interest in <u>getting out of</u>
<u>Vacant Attic Nursing Home.</u> Starfreak Command is always deeply concerned with the opinions of its underlings. You can be assured that my staff and I are giving every consideration to this matter. Please accept this handy pocket calendar with my best wishes.

Sincerely,
Admiral E.J. Cahoots

Enclosure: 12-month pocket calendar

Dear Jean-Lucy,
    Hey, guy, how's it going? I got your letter when my ship stopped in at Starbase 773 for an oil change. We had to pick up the letter personally 'cause there was postage due.
    I'd love to help get you out of your predicament, old buddy, but politically it's a little sticky right now,

especially since I'm about a year away from retirement myself and I don't want to screw that up by crossing Admiral Less' path, you know?

So I'll have to take a pass on your suggestion that I fly over to drop a futon torpedo on your nursing home's head office. But I'll be sure to stop by for a visit if I'm ever in your sector.

Live Long and Profit,
Capt. Chuck Vaguer

Listen, Smirk,

I know what you're up to. Writing from the nursing home under Capt. Ricardo's name is such a dumb stunt that I'm insulted you thought I'd fall for it.

Admiral Ruth Less

Dear Jean-Lucy,

It was good to hear from you again. I trust that our ongoing correspondence gives meaning to your days in the nursing home. It sounds as if you're becoming resigned to your situation. As you say, the bright side is that you no longer have the stress of making decisions, except for the tough task of choosing from selections on the dining hall menu. Perhaps one of the aides could help you with that.

I'm sending a bottle of our newest wine. The grapes in our vineyard are exceptional this year. Therefore, rather than wasting them on wine, we're eating them. This new wine is made of fermented tangerine peels. Nevertheless, I hope you enjoy it. Remember to drink it slowly since this is the real thing and not that simpahol stuff. You don't want to get soused. On the other hand, considering where you're living, you might as well guzzle it.

Your brother,
Rodney Ricardo

Dear Jean-Lucy Ricardo,
   I got your letter saying that you're stuck in the nursing home under a mistaken identity and that nobody in Starfreak believes you. However, I believe you. This is just the sort of dumb situation I always expected you to land in. Anybody who'd willingly spread fertilizer with his bare hands is going to come to a bad end—that's what I always say.
   It sounds like you have a lot of time on your hands, so I'm enclosing a gardening project to give you something to do. It's a Chia Pet. Just add water and it grows. I think you can handle it.

Sincerely,
Toothby the Gardener

Dear Commander Wilson Piker:
   What a surprise to hear from one of my former students. When did you learn to read and write? Certainly not in my classroom.
   You asked me to help you get out of the nursing home you're in, but I think that's a bad idea. In fact, considering your intelligence level, I think they're doing the galaxy a favor by keeping you locked up.

Sincerely,
Mrs. Crayon
Frozen Pipes Elementary School
Valdez, Alaska

Deanna baby,

It was really far-out to get your letter. So the nursing home guys think you're us, huh? That's pretty funny. I mean, not ha-ha funny, but weird funny.

I'm too busy to help you out right now, but if there's ever a lull in the babe situation here, I'll definitely see what I can do.

Ciao,
Jim Smirk

Dear Smartalecsander:

As your father, I am very concerned with the report card I just received from your teacher on the *Endocrine*. She wrote in the margin of the card that you are now the class bully. I expected more of you, young man. You should be the *ship's* bully by now. Get with it!

Wart

Dear Westerly,

My dear, dear son, I am writing to you on a matter of utmost urgency. All of us senior officers have been detained against our will in the Vacant Attic Nursing Home. Please tell someone in authority there at your Starfreak Academy Film School about our horrible predicament. All of my letters to others on the outside have gone unanswered. You're my last hope.

With motherly love,
Bev Flusher

Enclosure: your weekly allowance

Dear Mom,
   Thanks for the money. Please send more.
Love,
Westerly

Packing Slip

TO: Georgie LaForgery
RE: Repair of visor model #345A–7953D
COMMENTS:
   We have repaired your visor as requested. Seeing
that your return address is in the Vacant Attic Nursing Home, we have added a bifocal option at no extra
charge. We hope you enjoy your new visor.

Josie Whale
Repair manager, VisorCrafters

P.S. Regarding your other request: Sorry, but I can't
help spring you from the nursing home. I suggest
you check the Yellow Pages under SWAT teams and
find one that takes on freelance jobs.

Dear Miss Guano,
   I sincerely thank you for the fine cigars and wonderful letter. I did not know until today that the fed-
eral post office could deliver mail sent via time-travel
canister.
   You would hardly recognize San Francisco. It has
changed so much since your last visit, and horseless
carriages are everywhere.
   Nevertheless, some things never change. The android's discarded head remains in my household as
a remembrance of our exciting adventure; I have
been using it as a cuspidor. And I continue my practice of attending literary receptions and boring the

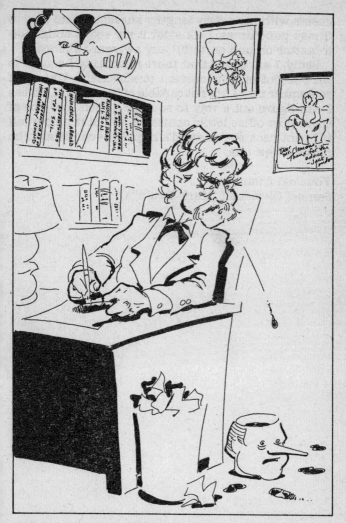

"The android's discarded head remains in my household as a remembrance of our exciting adventure."

guests with my overly lengthy anecdotes that lead to flimsy punchlines. I consider it my social obligation to natter on and on to fill any awkward silences.

Sadly, I am afraid that there is nothing I can do to get you out of your current predicament. You must remember that I am not capable of time travel, unless I can figure out a way to squeeze myself into one of these post office letter canisters. Would it help at all if I sent back the android's head? It sounds as if he needs a new one.

Your old friend,
Samuel Clemens ("Mark Twain")

8

A Hunka Hunka Burnin' 'Droid

Q-TIP STOOD IN THE WINGS, his gaze swiveling back and forth between Dacron, who was doing his Elvis schtick in the spotlight, and the mob of fans out in the audience. Dacron was playing the planet of Wilma-7 as part of his concert tour, and the show had started to heat up.

During this stretch of appearances, touted as the Resurrection Tour, Q-Tip had noticed a curious phenomenon. Every concert had a point at which the crowd's frenzy reached critical mass. It usually occurred about three-quarters of the way through the show, when the excitement level cranked up to a new plateau, the screams of the audience battered the stage like ocean waves, and a flash fire of hysteria spread through the auditorium.

At that point, people would do crazy things. Depending on what planet the tour was playing and the type of aliens in the audience, the fans might rush the stage, or tear their hair and clothes, or start throwing things, or faint, or begin speaking in tongues. Occasionally some of the aliens would metamorphose into other life forms or start eating each other.

Q-Tip surveyed the scene and speculated that tonight's concert had just about reached that breaking point.

He was right. A minute later, from one of the front rows, a pair of panties came sailing toward the stage. It looked like tonight would be a UFO night.

The panties triggered a deluge of flying objects. All were

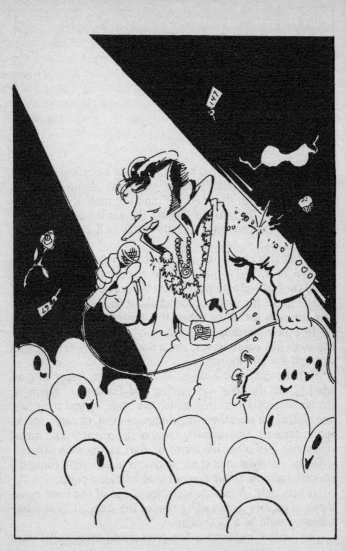

Dacron was playing the planet of Wilma-7.

gifts that the fans had brought in a desperate attempt to make some sort of connection with their idol. The air filled with their love offerings. Roses, handmade sweaters, jewelry and baked goods were rocketed at the stage. Dacron dodged them as gracefully as he could and kept on singing even after a schaum torte grazed his shoulder, leaving a streak of strawberry filling.

A stagehand standing beside Q-Tip clucked his tongue in disapproval. "All that good food going to waste," he said. "And throwing it at *him* yet. He doesn't look like he needs it."

"Hey, watch your mouth," Q-Tip snapped. "That's my boy out there."

Q-Tip knew as well as anyone that Dacron's waistline had expanded significantly from the grind of road touring. The greasy take-out food they often ate and other indulgences of the rock-'n'-roll lifestyle had already transformed the early Dacron into the late Dacron.

Yet criticism of the android was intolerable to Q-Tip, who lived vicariously through Dacron's superstardom. It was the kind of popularity that Q-Tip could never seem to achieve on his own, despite his omnipotence.

When Dacron finally left the stage at the conclusion of the concert, he was dripping with perspiration. "Man, it's a nuthouse out there," he panted as Q-Tip draped a towel around his neck and accompanied him down the backstage corridors to his dressing room.

"You really got them going tonight," Q-Tip exclaimed. "Isn't it a rush to feel all those people going crazy over you?"

"Ah dunno," Dacron said. "At first it was, but now ah just feel sorta...empty."

"A lot of performers would give their right arm to be in your position," Q-Tip reminded him.

"How about if ah give muh right arm to get *out* of muh position? Ah can unscrew it for yuh right now," Dacron moped. Then, under Q-Tip's stern gaze, he backed off a little. "Ah'm sorry, Colonel," he said. "Ah don't mean to be ungrateful. Ah know you're doin' a great job of steerin' muh career an' all, but it's jus' gettin' so crazy lately. All ah can think about is muh pals back at the Vacant Attic, and how much ah miss 'em, and how ah should be doin' somethin' to get 'em out of there. Muh mama would've wanted me to help 'em—if ah'd ever had a mama."

"You wouldn't be happy on that little hick planet," Q-Tip told him. "Your place is here in the big time. And there's more to come. I was going to save this for later, but I'll tell you now, just to cheer you up: I got a call today from the Ed Sullen show. They want you to be on the show this Saturday night! Isn't that great?"

Dacron knew that Q-Tip had been angling for this appearance, which represented the peak of his career to date. But to Dacron, greater fame only meant that he was ensnared even deeper in the celebrity web that now seemed so cumbersome.

"That's wunnerful, Colonel," Dacron said with as much enthusiasm as he could muster.

They turned the final corner down the hall to Dacron's dressing room. "Oh, no," Dacron groaned. "Not more groupies." About a dozen flashy women were clustered around the dressing room door, waiting for him.

"Too tired for a little feminine companionship?" Q-Tip asked, seeming disappointed that this vicarious pleasure was about to fall through.

"Ah may be fully functional, Colonel, but even ah have muh limits," Dacron replied, wearily rubbing his eyes with the towel.

"All right, then," Q-Tip conceded, escorting him through the crowd and into the dressing room, leaving the women outside.

The dressing room was arranged just as Dacron's contract specified. There was a buffet table with a six-pack of crankcase oil, several bags of Manny's Oat Bran Tortilla Chips, and a bowl of M&M candies with the green ones removed. One wall held a Snap-On Tools calendar with a boudoir photograph of

O-rings alluringly arranged on velvet. Light bulbs throughout the room heated up, spreading the scent of the Essence of Silicon cologne that had been sprayed on them.

Dacron sat in front of his dressing table and stared dully at his reflection in the mirror. "Yuh know," he said, "lately when ah look in the mirruh, ah get scared. There's no soul behind muh eyes."

"So what?" Q-Tip scoffed. "Like you had a soul before?"

"Ah did," Dacron protested. "And ah had a purpose in mah life when ah was on the ship. Ah used t' sit all day punchin' those buttons on mah console and sneakin' a peak at mah soap operas when the captain was off the Bridge. It was a good ol' time. Now ah'm on the road, and half the time ah don't even know which city ah'm in, an' it's just one gig after anothuh—"

"Oh, knock it off," Q-Tip snapped. "You performers are all alike. You'll do anything to get to the top, but then once you're there, all you can do is complain." Q-Tip adopted a whiny voice to imitate the litany of rock-star complaints: " 'Life on the road is so hard.' 'All they want to hear is the old hits, not my new songs.' 'Nobody knows how rough it is to spend a full two hours singing each night.' 'I want to be back home.' "

"Well, ah *do* wanna be back home!" Dacron said, flashing an uncharacteristic show of temper. "Or at least, back with muh friends at the Vacant Attic."

"Forget it!" Q-Tip snarled. "I told you before, we are not cutting short this tour. I didn't bring you this far to have you flake out on me. Especially now that we've snared a spot on the Sullen show." He and Dacron glared at each other, and Q-Tip added, "You know, your moodiness is making this tour a real drag. Snap out of it, will you?"

Q-Tip gestured at the dressing room door, then flicked his wrist and disappeared in a flash of light.

Dacron checked the door immediately. Just as he'd expected, Q-Tip had locked him in. He flung himself onto the couch and sulked for awhile; then he remembered that his secret stash was still hidden in the closet in a small suitcase.

Dacron opened the case and surveyed its contents, an array of android pharmaceutical software that helped him cope with the stress of his new life. There were uppers: various cleanup utilities that helped him get going in the morning. There were downers: Lotus spreadsheets he ran just before bedtime to help him sleep. And there were hallucinogens for the times he really needed to get away from it all. His favorite was a screen-saver program with a Lava Lite motif that projected itself against his closed eyelids.

Lately he'd become dangerously dependent on all of them, but he blamed it on the pressures of the road. Besides, he knew he could stop anytime. He just didn't want to.

After loading the Lava Lite screen-saver, Dacron lounged on the sofa. Immediately his muscles relaxed as the program worked its magic. His whirling thoughts started to settle down, and he pictured himself moving far away from the hassles of the tour. He dreamed of building a mansion where he could get away from it all. He'd make it into a palace, and it would become his own private retreat. He could call it Spaceland.

Back at Juven Isle, Cmdr. Crisco lurked in the bushes next to the log flume ride. He was casing the joint to figure out the best way to gain control of the water of the Fountain of Youth. That would let him get started on the second half of his mission: to build a trans-planetary pipeline that would deliver the water to Starfreak Command.

Crisco's return to the planet from the Vacant Attic had been delayed by a minor crisis involving his son, Joke. Smiles O'Brine, filling in for his wife Kookoo as a substitute teacher, had recommended that Joke undergo a psychological screening for Westerly Flusher Syndrome, a progressive disorder of the wimp nodes. Luckily, the evaluation turned out to be reassuring: the shrink told Crisco that Joke would probably

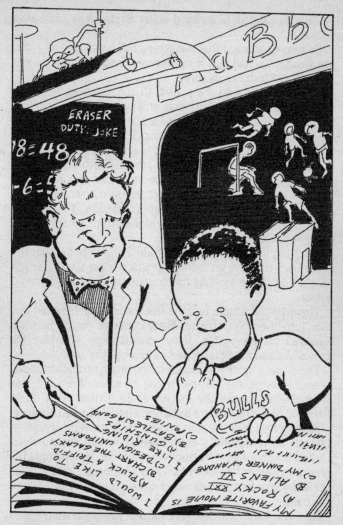

O'Brine had recommended Joke undergo a psychological screening for Westerly Flusher Syndrome.

be okay as long as he avoided active Bridge duty until after puberty.

Crisco was grateful that everything had turned out all right, but the detour had cost him precious time, and now he was chafing to finish his mission.

Upon his return to the planet, Crisco had been surprised to see that the theme park was still operating even though he'd taken Smirk & Co. to the Vacant Attic some time ago. He had assumed that once the ringleaders were gone, the whole park would shut down. But that hadn't happened. The place was going full blast. It was jammed with visitors, and there were plenty of employees around, too—far too many to allow Crisco to singlehandedly take over Juven Isle.

So he conducted a covert operation, sneaking through the island's plastic foliage and trying to determine where all this water was coming from.

Studying the layout, Crisco couldn't help noticing that the water truly did have an anti-aging effect. Rider after rider got off the log flume looking much younger than when they'd got on.

The artificial jungle became thicker as he penetrated farther into the phony island. Hefty canes of plastic bamboo hindered his every step. Ropey plastic vines ensnared his ankles. A canopy of plastic leaves blocked the sunlight.

There was a quick movement in the brush up ahead. Crisco peered through the foliage, trying to determine what was there. Failing to see the motion again, Crisco crept in its direction, ducking under a thick branch that blocked his view.

As Crisco pushed the branch aside, he felt a weird sensation against his neck, and a cold, slippery weight draped itself around his shoulders. Instinctively he froze. Moving only his eyes, he managed to determine, to his horror, that a huge tropical snake had just slithered down onto him from one of the trees.

Now don't panic, Crisco told himself as his stomach began doing the Twist. *Stay cool and think your way out of this, man. Figure out what kind of snake this is so you'll know how to deal with it. Is it a boa constrictor that's going to squeeze the breath out of you? Or is it a poisonous type that will sink its huge fangs into your cheek? Or maybe a garter snake that will spit in your eye and blind you? Or an eel that's going to drag you into the water and drown you? That's it—nice and cool . . .*

The rustling in the brush just ahead started up again, much louder this time. Crisco's skin crawled as he imagined the snake becoming spooked by the noise and killing him in an instant.

A young man pushed his way out of the foliage toward Crisco. His uniform had JUVEN ISLE SECURITY stitched on its pocket. "Can I help you, sir?" he inquired.

Crisco, still frozen like a statue, gestured wildly with his eyes to indicate the snake draped around his shoulders. The young man's expression registered surprise, but he recovered quickly. Nodding to Crisco, he whispered, "African Bamboozle Snake. Very poisonous. We'll have to take him to the park's kennel and knock him out with the sleeping-dart gun." The young man reached for Crisco's hand to lead him out of the brush.

Crisco whimpered as loudly as he dared, terrified to move from the spot.

"It's okay," continued the security guard in a whisper. "The snake will rest on your shoulders as long as you don't make any sudden movements."

Something—perhaps the look of serenity on the young man's Oriental features—inspired a smidgen of confidence in Crisco. Or maybe it was the fact that he had no choice. Whatever the reason, he followed ever so cautiously as the security guard led him out of the jungle surrounding Juven Isle.

They left the island and continued through the park. The trip down the pedestrian mall was a nightmare. Youngsters crowded near Crisco to see and touch the snake draped around his shoulders, while Crisco tried to warn them off with stern looks and ineffective finger-waving. The snake seemed to have fallen asleep and was apparently oblivious of the commotion, though every so often it shifted position an inch or so, striking terror into Crisco's heart.

Finally, after what seemed an eternity, they reached a cluster of small office buildings. Crisco followed as the young man proceeded to an inner room. "Here he is, Captain Smirk," called the young guard. Dimly, in the midst of his terror, Crisco wondered about the significance of this greeting and of the name the guard had spoken.

There in the inner office, another young man sat with his feet propped cockily on his desk. He studied Crisco with a wry smile. The young man's amusement, his lack of surprise at the menacing snake, even his sweatshirt that read KISS ME, I'M SENTIENT—it all began to seem surreal to Crisco. He wondered if he was having another one of his pepperoni nightmares.

"Thank you, Mr. Zulu. Sit down, Commander Crisco," said the young man, grinning, as he gestured toward the guest chair. Fleetingly Crisco wondered how this stranger knew his name. The youngster gazed at him steadily as Crisco, staring straight ahead and holding his shoulders rigid to avoid disturbing the snake, maneuvered his rear into the chair and unwittingly sat on a cardboard pizza carton someone had left there.

"Can I get you anything?" the young man offered. He reached into a small refrigerator, retrieved several beverage cans, and brought them to Crisco's side of the desk. "Soda? Fruit drink?" Crisco, afraid even to shake his head, moved his eyes from side to side.

"I know," said the young man. "Maybe you'd like something for your *snake*!" To Crisco's horror, the youngster grabbed the snake and began twisting his hands around its body.

Sheer fright knocked the breath out of Crisco, and for an instant he blacked out. When he came to, he saw that the young man and the security guard were laughing hysterically. The snake was stretched out on the desk, belly-up, motionless—and even from a few feet away Crisco could see the legend stamped on its underside: MADE IN TAIWAN.

Overcome with laughter, the young men fell down and rolled on the floor, hooting and howling. Crisco felt the slow burn of the realization that he'd just been scammed.

When the other two finally caught their breath, they gave each other a bear hug. "Right on, Security Chief!" exclaimed the sweatshirted youngster. The other left the room. The one with the sweatshirt climbed back into his desk chair, brushing the dust of the floor off his sleeves.

"Whew! That was classic!" he exclaimed. He extended a hand, and the stunned Crisco reflexively reached out to shake it. "Welcome to Juven Isle," said the young man. "I'm Captain James T. Smirk. Now maybe you'd like to tell me why you were sneaking around in my plastic jungle, hmmmm?"

Dacron rolled over in bed and moaned as he unwillingly drifted into wakefulness. Sunlight sneaked past the edges of the thick drapes hanging over the window of his hotel luxury suite. Judging from the intensity of the sun, the time was well past dawn, but to Dacron's groggy circuits it felt like the middle of the night.

Vaguely he recalled that his entourage had arrived in the city sometime after midnight. They'd taken rooms in a hotel near the studio where Dacron would appear on the Ed Sullen show that evening. There'd been a party in his room—that much Dacron remembered—and when everyone had finally left, he'd been too keyed up to sleep. He'd loaded a game program into his head just for kicks. Everything after that was just a blank; Dacron speculated that the game must have had a bug in it.

Wham! The door burst open and slammed against the adjacent wall. Q-Tip stormed into the room. His irate expression made it clear that he'd chosen this unusual—for him—method of entry to create the biggest possible ruckus.

"Why are you still in bed?" Q-Tip demanded. He wrenched open the drapes, staggering Dacron with a blast of sunlight.

"It's five o'clock in the afternoon!" Q-Tip barked. "You're due at the Ed Sullen studio in less than an hour!"

Groaning, Dacron tried to pull the covers over his head, but Q-Tip stomped over to the bedside and yanked the covers off.

"Look at you," Q-Tip sneered. "You've really let yourself go. There's nothing more disgusting than an android with a pot belly."

Dacron shivered, curling up against the mattress and covering his head with one of the Heartbreak Hotel's satin pillows.

"Well, get up!" Q-Tip ordered.

"Ah cain't," Dacron whimpered.

"You miserable bucket of bolts!" Q-Tip raged. "This is your big chance! Don't you realize that you'll be the first android Sullen's ever had on the show? You can be a credit to your species!" Dacron tried to avoid him by turning over, but Q-Tip flashed to the other side of the bed and thrust his face next to Dacron's. "After being on the Sullen show," Q-Tip said, "you'll be able to call the shots in your career. You'll play all the big venues—Vegas, Venus, Vega, even the Vela system. Your face will be known from Maine to blue Hawaii."

"Ah don't cay-are," Dacron whined. "Ah wanna be back with muh pals, the people who love me tender. Ah'm tahred of all this high livin'. Ah never was much of a high livuh t' begin with. Don't make me go on, Colonel. Don' be cruel."

"Surely you can't be serious," said Q-Tip with a hint of trembling in his voice. "You wouldn't turn down a chance to do—*Ed Sullen*."

"Yes, ah would," Dacron insisted, rolling over onto his back and folding his arms across his chest in defiance. "And you cain't make me."

They both knew this was true. Once before, when Dacron was suffering a similar nervous breakdown tinged with rebelliousness, Q-Tip had physically forced him through the mechanics of his stage show. The result was patently fake, and the fans had actually booed him.

Q-Tip knew that to try a similar maneuver for this Sullen appearance would be disastrous. Dacron would bomb on intergalaxywide live TV, and instead of the vicarious pleasure Q-Tip anticipated, he'd endure vicarious embarrassment. Just imagining the scene made Q-Tip feel all shook up.

"Dacron, please." Q-Tip grasped the android's arm. "You know how much this means to me. This would be the ultimate thrill. I simply must feel that excitement from the audience one more time. Remember, you owe me one. I'm responsible for bringing you here out of nowhere from your job in the ghetto of Ricardo's starship. Please do the show. Please!"

Dacron sulked for a few moments longer, then allowed, "Well, maybe. But only if you promise me somethin'."

"Anything. Anything," Q-Tip answered eagerly.

"Promise me that after this ah'll stop tourin' for a while and go back to muh friends," said Dacron. "And that you'll help me get 'em out of that nursin' home and back into our ship."

"I promise," Q-Tip assured him.

Wearily, Dacron rose from the bed. Q-Tip sighed with relief, then headed for the bathroom. "You get your stage clothes on," he ordered, "while I'm heating up the hot rollers for your hair."

Once he'd gotten over the shock of the snake scare, Crisco began to relax in Smirk's office, and as the two of them talked, Crisco even got to like Smirk. And there was much to like, for Smirk was at his most charming: serving soft drinks and snack chips, chatting about Starfreak, drawing out stories about Crisco's past, and revealing candidly that Crisco had transported the wrong crew to the Vacant Attic Nursing Home. Smirk even described what it felt like when he and his crew transformed from old geezers into young punks after they'd captured the Fountain of Youth.

Yet through it all Crisco sensed that Smirk wasn't about to let him walk out the door unrestricted. There was still the little matter of who controlled the fountain. And it was clear that right now that control resided firmly in Smirk's hands.

The conversation turned to the hardships of Starfreak life. Smirk commiserated with Crisco over the loss of his wife and revealed that he himself had once lost an adult son. "Not that Starfreak Command ever really cared," Smirk mused. "You wouldn't believe the paperwork I had to wade through just to get some honest-to-goodness embalming fluid for him. They were gonna use peanut oil, for Pete's sake."

"It's hard to imagine you having a grown son," Crisco murmured, studying Smirk's unlined face.

"Yeah, I suppose," said Smirk, rubbing his hand over his smooth cheeks. "But I was old once, just like you."

Crisco stared at the far corner and revealed bitterly, "Starfreak gave me a hard time, too, after my wife died. They said an officer with my ranking was only allotted thirty minutes of bereavement time with pay. I'm still trying to get the rest of my paycheck for that week."

"They'll put the screws to ya every chance they get," Smirk said with a world-weary shake of his young head. He seemed lost in thought for a few minutes. Then he shook himself out of his reverie and remarked, "So you say Starfreak Command ordered you to take my Fountain of Youth water and pipe it back to them?"

"What?" Crisco, too, emerged from his trip down memory lane. He made a face. "Starfreak? Aw, heck, screw 'em."

Smirk grinned at Crisco's insolence, then predicted, "Yeah, but if you come back empty-handed, they'll just send somebody else. Eventually, somebody's gonna take over my fountain."

"That's true," Crisco concluded reluctantly. His expression made it clear that he no longer thought this was a fair course of action.

"Unless..." said Smirk, mulling over some possibility.

"Unless what?" Crisco prompted.

"Well, you could still build your pipeline," Smirk said,

seeming to make up a plan as he went along. "That would take the heat off both of us."

"Then you'd be willing to pump some water to Starfreak?" Crisco asked.

"I could," Smirk went on. "Nobody's saying how *much* water, if you catch my meaning. Like, you don't know what the daily production of the fountain is, right?"

"Right," Crisco agreed, catching on.

"So if I send, say twenty-thousand youtholiters a day to Starfreak, they're gonna assume that's the total volume of water coming out of the fountain. And if I also set you up with a steady supply of bottled water for resale, and keep the rest of the fountain water running through Juven Isle, no one's the wiser, right?"

"Right," Crisco said, clearly pleased at the thought of cheating Starfreak out of a major portion of the spoils.

Smirk added, "Especially not Ricardo and his crew, livin' the high life over there in the Vacant Attic, 'cause you and I aren't about to tell anyone who they really are, right?"

"Right!" Crisco exclaimed.

"This calls for a toast," Smirk declared. He opened his refrigerator and pulled out two souvenir bottles of fountain water. "What d'ya wanna drink to?" he asked, handing one bottle to Crisco.

Crisco responded, "Let's drink to you and your crew—forever young." They clinked their bottles together and chug-a-lugged with relish.

9

Finis

"**A**LL RIGHT, CLASS, here we go. Now, has everybody got their little looms out? Good." As the instructor opened another session of the Potholder Weaving class, Capt. Ricardo studied the small square metal frame on the table in front of him. A worried frown creased his face.

During the past month, he and his classmates had spent two class periods each week stretching loops of doubleknit fabric over their frames. Now came the tricky part: weaving the other half of the loops over and under the original loops, at right angles, to form the fabric of the potholder.

Capt. Ricardo had been dreading this moment. This next step required the use of a latch hook and sounded dreadfully complicated. And it intensified the constant danger that a loop of fabric, stretched to its full length, might somehow work one end loose of the frame and turn into a deadly missile.

Ricardo's universe had definitely shrunk since the day he and his crew first checked into the Vacant Attic. Initially they'd remained in the nursing home against their will, since no one from the outside would come to their rescue.

But after some time, almost without noticing it, they became resigned to their situation. Eventually, nursing home life brought out the bland vanilla side of them all, and they even grew to like it at the Vacant Attic.

The nursing home was calm and peaceful. Everybody got along so well. There was no backbiting, no bickering—in fact, no character conflict whatsoever.

Soon they dropped their letter-writing campaign aimed at getting someone to rescue them, and they settled into their assumed identity as Capt. Smirk and crew. Their placid routines plodded along with the nursing home's cheery activity schedule: Bingo on Monday, arm exercise class on Wednesday, "Go Fish" card tournaments on Thursday, and cookie-and-milk socials on Sunday afternoons.

For crewmembers who desired additional challenges, the Vacant Attic offered plenty of classes in various skills, like the art of potholder weaving which Capt. Ricardo was now trying to master.

"Pick up your latch hook and place a loop of fabric on it like this," said the instructor. Warily Ricardo followed her example.

Suddenly someone appeared in the chair next to him. It was Q-Tip.

"My, my, *mon capitalist*," said Q-Tip, studying Ricardo's potholder frame with a sardonic grin, "I never dreamed you were so artistic."

Ricardo glared at him and set down his latch hook. "Q-Tip, you mustn't appear and disappear so suddenly," he said. "You're likely to give one of these people a heart attack."

"Say, who are you?" the instructor demanded, staring at Q-Tip. "Have you signed up for this session?"

Q-Tip ignored her and asked Ricardo, "Well, aren't you curious about why I came here?"

"Not really," said Ricardo, squirming as the entire class turned to stare at them. "Why don't you leave before you get me in trouble?"

"Oh, dear, dear, dear," Q-Tip said, *tsk-tsk*ing his tongue in mock exasperation. "How little it takes to rile you these days." He picked up a fabric loop, stretched it to its full length, and aimed it threateningly at Ricardo.

"All right," Ricardo said, nervously eyeing Q-Tip's weapon, "why *did* you come here, Q-Tip?"

"So glad you asked," Q-Tip said, lowering the loop. "I've

brought your boy back." He snapped his fingers, and Dacron appeared next to them in all his rockabilly glory.

"Hullo, Cap'n," said Dacron. "It's so good to see y'all again."

"And there's more," Q-Tip continued, "but I don't want to go into that here. Let's move to your room where we can have a little privacy." Q-Tip snapped his fingers again, and the three of them instantly transported to Ricardo's small bedroom.

Another snap of Q-Tip's fingers, and the rest of Ricardo's crew appeared in the room also. They blinked, surprised by the sudden change in their surroundings. Q-Tip had snatched them from a variety of activities that were reflected in the clothing they wore. Troit and Piker sat there in wet bathing suits, having been taken from a water aerobics session. Wart and Georgie were wearing smocks from their watercolor painting class. And Dr. Flusher and Guano were still in their bathrobes.

Seeing that Dacron had returned, the others gathered around him with hugs and exclamations. Q-Tip tapped his foot impatiently until the commotion died down; then he announced, "You'll all be happy to know that at the request of your homesick android, I'm here to take you away from this wasteland of boredom."

The crewmembers drooped. A blanket of silence hung over them.

"Well, hey, ever'body!" Dacron exclaimed, trying to drum up some enthusiasm. "Don't y'all wanna go back to the ship and get out of here?"

The silence stretched on. A couple of people shrugged their shoulders. A few cleared their throats nervously. There was shuffling of feet.

"What's the matter with you people?" Q-Tip demanded. "I didn't expect a ticker-tape parade, but at least you could show a *little* gratitude. This is what you've been waiting for, isn't it?"

Capt. Ricardo spoke up. "We did want to be rescued, some time ago," he allowed, "but lately that prospect has seemed rather remote, and I guess we've all become resigned to our situation. We even rather like it here."

Q-Tip's expression hardened with anger and disgust. "Like it?" he hissed. "You like it here?"

One by one, the others nodded. Dacron looked disappointed but said nothing.

"Of all the . . . you humans are just . . . " Q-Tip sputtered. "How utterly, utterly . . . *boring!*" he spat out, as if it were the worst insult he could muster.

"This is no fun at all anymore!" Q-Tip went on. "Even you!"—he pointed at Dacron—"You're getting to be a real drag. You're no longer fit to be The King." With a wave of his hand, Q-Tip transformed Dacron back into his old strait-laced, un-potbellied self.

"I'm leaving," Q-Tip concluded. "It'd be more fun to pick on a group of insurance actuaries than to hang around you people any longer!" With a flash, he disappeared.

"Well," Capt. Ricardo said. "Let's all get back to what we were doing, shall we?"

That night, Dacron began the transition to nursing-home life by giving another concert for the residents. Though he was pretty much back in his android mode, his circuits still contained trace imprints of show-biz patterns, and this concert was his way of livening up the somnolent nursing-home atmosphere.

Onstage, Dacron's movements were a lot stiffer and jerkier than in his Elvis days, and his singing voice had returned to its falsetto range; but he still had a spark of the old fire left in him, and his ad libs were much more to the point than they'd been before.

"My, what an exuberant crowd," he remarked at one point. "Are you all aware of the correct manner in which to rock-'n'-roll?" And later: "I would like to dedicate this number to a delightful young woman I met after one of my concerts. I shall never forget how her manual dexterity relaxed my severe case of post-concert bodily tension." And still later, glancing offstage as he wiped his sleeve against his forehead, "May I have a glass of crankcase oil, please? This activity is severely dehydrating."

Unfortunately, although Dacron's ad libs were better, overall his act was much less polished without Q-Tip's guidance. He'd put his belt buckle on backwards. His hair had lost its body; now, parted in the middle, it hung limply over his forehead as if he were emulating Shemp of the Three Stooges. And Dacron had made an unfortunate choice in the order of his songs, choosing "Are You Lonesome Tonight?" as his closing number.

Up to that point the place was rocking, but this ballad draped a melancholy mood over the nursing home residents. They truly were lonesome tonight, and every night, for their nearest relatives lived on other planets and rarely came to visit. By the time Dacron finished the song, a fog of longing had settled over the audience. He left the stage to a smattering of applause.

The nurses, nurses' aides and other workers were dismayed by this turn of events. They began clapping and calling, "Encore! Encore!" When Dacron failed to return to the stage, they began stomping their feet and pounding the walls. A few of them borrowed residents' walkers and rhythmically thumped them against the floor.

Capt. Ricardo went backstage to see if he could persuade Dacron to extend the concert and pacify the workers. A few minutes later Ricardo emerged onto the stage, holding up his hands for silence. He approached the microphone as the crowd quieted to hear his announcement.

"I'm sorry, but the concert really is over," Ricardo told them. "Dacron has left the building."

"Well done, Commander Crisco, well done," said Admiral Less, leaning back in her chair and regarding with approval the officer sitting on the other side of her huge power desk.

"Thank you," Crisco responded, trying not to stare at Less'

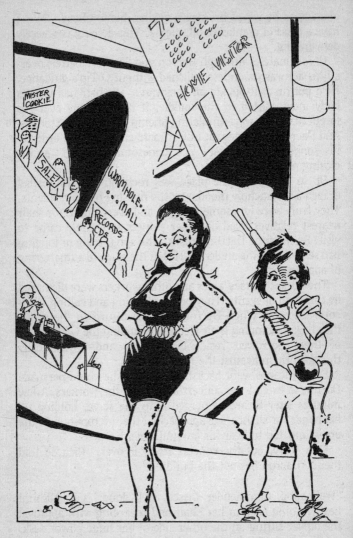

"This station is sort of wild and woolly."

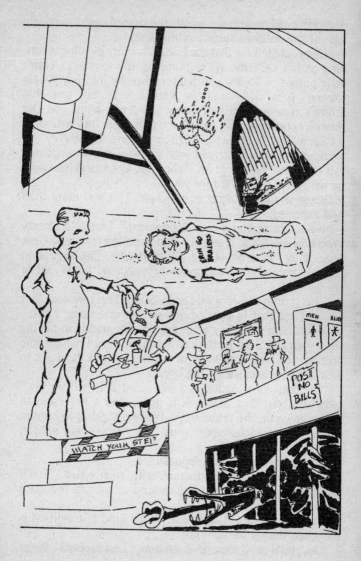

daggerlike red fingernails, which she rubbed absentmindedly against the polished surface of the desk.

"My people tell me that the trans-planetary pipeline is running at full capacity. We're pumping the fountain's entire daily output of 20,000 youtholiters directly into our supply towers," Less said. "And the Vacant Attic staff says that Smirk's crew has adjusted nicely to nursing-home life. Did they give you any trouble when you took them into custody?"

"Some, but I handled it," Crisco responded smoothly.

"Starfreak is very pleased with the way you've conducted this mission," Less went on. "The High Command has come up with a special reward for you."

Crisco straightened up in his chair. This was more than he'd expected.

"We're giving you a new assignment," Less told Crisco. "You'll be in charge of a space station on the frontier—Geek Space Nine, in orbit of the planet Badger. The federation recently booted the Carcinogen occupational forces out of there.

"This station is sort of wild and woolly," Less revealed, "but you can use that to your advantage. For one thing, I know your son hasn't had any adult female role models in his life since your wife died. Well, Geek Space Nine has a holographic brothel, so there are plenty of females around. It ought to provide some balance for the boy.

"The security situation is a bit . . . unruly, shall we say," Less went on, "but Starfreak is giving you a free hand to clamp down on the crime wave. We're not going to require you to file an official report every time you fire your phaser, if you catch my drift."

"Yes, ma'am," Crisco responded.

Admiral Less hesitated momentarily, then added, "You'll also notice that the Carcinogens kind of trashed the place before pulling out."

Crisco frowned with concern. "What kind of condition is the space station in, Admiral?"

"Oh, you'll get it fixed up in no time," Less breezed. "We're giving you plenty of expert help. Transporter Chief Smiles O'Brine is transferring there from the crew of the *Endocrine*—the new *Endocrine*, that is. He's prepared detailed engineering specs for sweeping up the pieces of the station's UltraFax and glueing them back together. And there's your first officer, who's a former Bridgeoran terrorist—she's very handy with explosives, I hear. You ought to be able to use that somehow. Every commander needs a good explosion now and then to keep the staff on their toes."

Less opened a file folder on her desktop. "Let's see about some of the others at the station . . . " she said, scanning a document. "There's a lieutenant—this duty roster says she's a 300-year-old slug in the body of a fashion model . . . huh, that oughta be interesting.

"Someone named Dodo," Less continued, reading aloud, "is the shape-shifting security officer. He keeps his department's expenses low by turning himself into a German Shepherd, a pair of handcuffs, a nightstick, or whatever he needs . . .

"There's a nightclub on the promenade, owned by a civilian Ferengi," Less went on, speaking to herself. "Gads, are we never going to shake these dratted Ferengi? They've become the houseflies of the galaxy."

Less read the roster in silence for a minute, her expression growing increasingly skeptical. Then, realizing Crisco was studying her, she concluded briskly, "Well, you get the drift." She snapped the personnel folder shut as if she feared Crisco would glimpse something revealing.

Crisco summoned a wan smile, fighting back the suspicion that his promotion was about to confirm the Peter Principle that employees always rise to their level of incompetence.

At Juven Isle Amusement Park, another happy day dawned. It couldn't help but be a happy day, for the Patent Office of the United Federation of Planets had just officially approved the park's application for a trademark on its slogan, "The Happiest Place in the Galaxy."

Capt. Smirk and six of that week's girlfriends boarded the Tower of Power ride in the center of the park. He'd commandeered the ride today for their private use. They were going to ride to the top of the tower and enjoy the view all day long as the round cabin revolved at its leisurely speed. They'd brought along a picnic lunch and a CD player to make the day complete.

"This is, like, too cool," one of the girls said as the cabin began climbing the tower. She opened the lid of the picnic cooler. "D'you wanna drink, Jim?"

"Sure, sweets," Smirk replied. "I'm dyin' of thirst. It's been at least half an hour since I've had a cola."

As she handed him the can of soda, Smirk plopped into one of the seats that faced the bank of windows overlooking the park. With his arms outstretched to the girls sitting on either side, he surveyed the grounds and felt a deep sense of satisfaction.

From his perch, Smirk could see the parking lot where their *Endocrine* was stored. Mr. Smock, he knew, would be busy monitoring the controls, keeping an eye on all vehicles approaching the planet, and maintaining the park's underground vacuum waste-disposal system.

From this height, no sound reached them, but Smirk glanced at the Migraine Bumper Cars building where Snotty was performing repairs today, and imagined he could hear the young engineer's frustrated rantings.

A long line of park visitors was already forming outside the first aid building. Smirk speculated that McCaw had once again posted his "The doctor is OUT" sign with a picture of a medic wielding a five-iron.

In one corner of the park, the Ferocious Ferris was spinning faster than ever. Smirk could just barely see the tiny form of Checkout beneath it, dodging seats as he continued his gum-scraping duties. Checkout claimed to be getting more adept at the task; now he only got struck by every tenth seat.

At the other end of the park, Smirk saw a few patrons

running out of the theater—apparently terrorized—and he figured that Yoohoo must have just taken the stage.

The newest thrill ride, Samurai Slicer, was up and running. Smirk knew that Zulu would be carefully monitoring his creation. As riders bounced on the rocking platform and tried to avoid the huge blades that randomly whooshed down at them from overhead, Zulu would keep a sharp lookout, ready to press the "Emergency Stop" button if there was a close call. So far the ride had had just a few fatalities, and these had only increased its reputation—there was always a two-hour wait in line to get on.

The girls on either side of Smirk began angling for his attention. He turned away from the window and flashed a stunning glance at each of them in turn.

One of them began feeding him grapes. The other whipped out a manicure set and began doing his nails.

Smirk relaxed in his chair and declared to no one in particular, "This is the life!"

An old battle cry popped into Smirk's head. Filled with jubilation that things had turned out so well, he proclaimed:

"These are, like, the voyages of the Starship *Endocrine*. Its mission: to, you know, cruise around the universe looking for totally cool situations to get into . . . to search the outskirts of the galaxy for hot babes . . . to, like, boldly go where nobody wanted to go before!"

Boldly go where nobody ever wanted to go before!

Leah Rewolinski's *Star Wreck* books—which parody everyone's favorite endlessly rerun TV series, not to mention everyone's favorite interminable number of movie sequels and everyone's favorite "next generation" spin-off—are turning the world—and the galaxy—on its collective pointed ear!

STAR WRECK: THE GENERATION GAP
_____ 92802-5 $3.99 U.S./$4.99 CAN.

STAR WRECK II: THE ATTACK OF THE JARGONITES
_____ 92737-1 $3.99 U.S./$4.99 CAN.

STAR WRECK III: TIME WARPED
_____ 92891-2 $3.99 U.S./$4.99 CAN.

STAR WRECK IV: LIVE LONG AND PROFIT
_____ 92985-4 $3.99 U.S./$4.99 CAN.

Publishers Book and Audio Mailing Service
P.O. Box 120159, Staten Island, NY 10312-0004
Please send me the book(s) I have checked above. I am enclosing $ _____ (please add $1.50 for the first book, and $.50 for each additional book to cover postage and handling. Send check or money order only—no CODs) or charge my VISA, MASTERCARD, DISCOVER or AMERICAN EXPRESS card.

Card number _____

Expiration date _____ Signature _____

Name _____

Address _____

City _____ State/Zip _____
Please allow six weeks for delivery. Prices subject to change without notice. Payment in U.S. funds only. New York residents add applicable sales tax.

SW 1/93

- If the mistake is in your favor, don't correct it.
- Cut people off in the middle of their sentences.
- Turn on your brights for oncoming traffic.
- Develop a convenient memory.
- Take personal calls during important meetings.
- Carve your name in picnic tables.
- Don't leave a message at the beep.
- Leave your supermarket cart on the street or in the parking lot.
- Ask her if the diamond ring is real.
- Before exiting the elevator, push all the buttons.

These and 502 more boorish, insensitive and socially obnoxious pointers for leading a simple, self-centered life may be found in

Life's Little Destruction Book
A Parody

A Stonesong Press Book by
Charles Sherwood Dane
Available from St. Martin's Press

LIFE'S LITTLE DESTRUCTION BOOK
Charles Sherwood Dane
_____ 92927-7 $5.99 U.S./$6.99 Can.

Publishers Book and Audio Mailing Service
P.O. Box 120159, Staten Island, NY 10312-0004
Please send me the book(s) I have checked above. I am enclosing $ _____ (please add $1.50 for the first book, and $.50 for each additional book to cover postage and handling. Send check or money order only—no CODs) or charge my VISA, MASTERCARD, DISCOVER or AMERICAN EXPRESS card.

Card number _____

Expiration date _____ Signature _____

Name _____

Address _____

City _____ State/Zip_____
Please allow six weeks for delivery. Prices subject to change without notice. Payment in U.S. funds only. New York residents add applicable sales tax.

LLDB 3/92